The Beginner's Guide

to

MEDICAL CANNABIS

Professor Michael P Barnes, MD, FRCP

Honorary Professor of Neurological Rehabilitation,
University of Newcastle

The Beginner's Guide to Medical Cannabis

ISBN print: 978-1-912798-06-3

ISBN e book: 978-1-912798-05-6

This book is dedicated to Alfie Dingley

and his family

BEFORE USING THE INFORMATION IN THIS BOOK

Always consult your own doctor before taking new medication or supplements or making any changes to your prescribed medical regime. The information contained in this book is not a substitute for such a consultation; it should not take the place of medical professional advice in any way and should not be treated as such.

Similarly, if you are seeking help for a child, you must first refer to their medical professional before changing their medication, introducing new medication or supplements.

There is a reference section at the back of this book where you can find information about the studies we mention. It's at the back so that the references don't take up too much footnote space on each page.

All prices and details correct at the time of publishing but as this is a fast-moving area, please check.

CONTENTS

INTRODUCTION

I first became interested in medical cannabis in the late 1990s. I was running clinics for people with multiple sclerosis (MS), in my role as consultant neurologist in the NHS. Many said they were using cannabis and finding it helpful both for their pain and their muscle spasms. I then asked all the patients as they came to the clinic about cannabis use, and most were prepared to tell me. It turned out that about 50 per cent of the patients were users. That made me think that there was something to this plant. Why, otherwise, would so many law-abiding citizens use an illegal product? Why would disabled people especially, take the risk of prosecution and expose themselves to the difficulties of obtaining the product?

Then, by chance, the first legal cannabis product began trials in the UK in 1999. This was Sativex made by the British drug company G W Pharmaceuticals who were founded a year earlier in 1998 and were the only drug company developing cannabis isolates. Through my role as a trustee of the Multiple Sclerosis Trust, I became involved in their studies as an independent expert and ultimately helped G W with the presentation of their trial data to the licensing authorities. In 2010, Sativex became the first legal cannabis product to be licensed in the UK and is used for relief of muscle spasms (spasticity) in multiple sclerosis (MS) and other conditions.

Then the National Institute for Health and Care Excellence (NICE), the National Health Service (NHS) department who publish guidelines on drug use, said that Sativex was not cost effective and should not be funded by the NHS. So, all went quiet for a while.

In May 2016, I was asked to write a resumé of the evidence of effectiveness of cannabis for the UK government's *All Party Parliamentary Group on Drug Policy Reform*. My daughter, Dr. Jennifer Barnes, and I did this, and I hope that our report helped to move the issue up the political agenda. Medical cannabis, in all its forms except smoking, was finally passed for use in the UK on 1 November 2018.

Since 2016, I have helped with the media campaign to have cannabis legalised for medical use and worked with some wonderful people like those at the charity End our Pain and Hannah Deacon, Alfie Dingley's mother. Alfie Dingley, age six, suffers with childhood epilepsy which did not respond well to conventional drugs. His parents took him to the Netherlands and found he did respond well to medical cannabis, although he wasn't allowed to bring the THC variety back to the UK as it wasn't legal. In June 2018, we managed to get Alfie the first ever UK license for cannabis to be used as a medicine.

I have now many hundreds of stories from people who have benefitted from cannabis for many conditions. No medicine is a cure-all, but there is no doubt that medical cannabis can help many people with many different conditions.

Some types of medical cannabis can be bought from health food shops without prescription, whilst other types have to be prescribed. You can self-medicate, taking capsules, oil, edibles or vaping, and it's not a medicine that needs to be injected. It's also kind to your stomach and is not addictive.

I am glad it is now legal for doctors to prescribe in the UK. We still have a long way to go in terms of persuading doctors to suggest it for their patients, but education will help there. Undoubtedly, the campaign has come far in a short period of time.

I hope this book is a helpful introduction to the versatile medicinal plant called cannabis.

Mike Barnes

Newcastle upon Tyne   March 2019

PART 1

CHAPTER 1

What is medical cannabis and what can it do?

A 'well-being' medicine

We're only just beginning to understand the full power of cannabis, even though it's been around for thousands of years. Cannabis improves symptoms and can cure some diseases, but it is best at symptom management rather than cure. It helps with sleep, anxiety, pain and appetite and can generally improve your quality of life. You could say that cannabis is a well-being medicine.

Look how it can help with pain management and with the side-effects caused by cancer treatment:

Cannabis has the ability to control pain so well, no matter what the cause, that 25 per cent of people taking strong opioid painkillers are able to replace them with medical cannabis[i]. In 2018, the Centers for Disease Control (CDC)[ii] in the US, reported that prescription opioids kill 49,000 people annually. In the UK, the Office for National Statistics[iii] reported in 2018 that around 4,000 people died after taking prescription opioids. Because of under-reporting, the true figures are likely to be much higher. Medical cannabis is a non-toxic alternative. This is tremendous news, but it is a point often missed by politicians, regulators and many medics.

As for cancer, according to a number of good quality scientific studies, cannabis will help not only with your pain, but also your nausea, your appetite and your anxiety. It can improve your mood, relaxes you and improves your sleep.

In other words, cannabis improves your quality of life. There is nothing wrong with that. In my view, that's medicine at its best — helping people when they need it most.

What is medical cannabis?
Medical cannabis comes from three different species of wild cannabis: sativa, indica and ruderalis. Sativa is from Latin and means cultivated, indica is Latin for 'of India' and ruderalis is the Latin meaning 'rubble', 'lump' or 'piece of bronze'.

The ruderal varieties emerge first in any wasteland — a bit like weeds that pop up anywhere, they bloom through the rubble — but on the pharmacy shelves, indica and sativa varieties are the most popular. Many growers combine the positive benefits of stimulating sativa and sedating indica into various hybrids.

Recreational drug or medicine?
Today, we think of cannabis more as a recreational drug, but that's a fairly recent development, for thousands of years, it was used mainly as medicine.

Those who use it as a recreational drug like the marijuana 'high' effects that it can have on the brain. These are euphoria and sedation and are caused by a psychoactive compound with an amazing Star Wars sounding name delta-9-tetrahydrocannabinol (THC). In medical cannabis, the THC content is heavily regulated and reduced to avoid unwanted side effects. Understandably, this makes us feel cautious when thinking about taking it as medicine. 'Will I end up walking round like a zombie or giggling uncontrollably?' With medical cannabis, this does not usually happen, and this book will explain why.

What's in a cannabis plant?

The cannabis plant is made up of around 100 compounds (cannabinoids), over 100 terpenes (aromatic compounds) and 20 flavonoids (pigments), all of which have medical properties. Scientists are working their way through the compounds and terpenes to see which does what and which is the most beneficial when it comes to our health. So far, they have identified two main compounds: cannabidiol (CBD) and THC. Four minor compounds have also been identified that are considered big hitters when it comes to our health.

The medicinal effects of cannabis have been known for generations, but we are only now trying to define what each individual component does, and which one causes what effect. Our ancestors knew instinctively what these were but in the 21st century, understandably, we want scientific proof.

Many of the studies into CBD, THC and the other cannabinoids found in cannabis, are in mice or rats, but that's where all the best research starts. There are human studies which have really positive results too, and more are in the pipeline.

What we know for sure is:

Cannabidiol (CBD) and Delta-9-tetrahydrocannabinol (THC)

CBD — Is non psychoactive and is useful in managing epilepsy, pain disorders, brain injury, neurological disorders, sleep

disorders, gastrointestinal disorders, mood, behaviour, and has anti-cancer properties

CBD is widely, and legally, available in many countries. It is often marketed as a food supplement, rather than a medicine as it contains over 100 compounds while most medicines tend to be based on one compound. In the UK, the **Medicines and Healthcare Products Regulatory Agency (MHRA)** states that all medicinal products must have a licence before they can be marketed as medicines. This does not mean that CBD is not effective, and the British government says that specialists can prescribe it.

According to many studies:

- It has an anti-anxiety effect. In 2011, Brazilian researchers[iv] conducted a double-blind placebo-controlled trial to confirm this.

- It is strongly anti-convulsant and has become important in the management of drug resistant epilepsies, particularly in children.

- In 2012, researchers at the University of Milan, Italy[v], discovered that CBD seems to have an anti-cancer effect, at least in certain specific human cancers. The *Molecular Cancer Therapeutics*[vi] journal published a study in 2011 showing that it was effective in the fight against breast cancer.

- In 2000, the National Institute of Mental Health[vii] (NIMH) in the US, the government's research centre, acknowledges that CBD is neuroprotective and helps to stabilise and prevent damage to the nervous system after insults like stroke or traumatic brain injury. They have even taken out a patent recognising that fact.

- CBD is a useful painkiller. Many medical journals have published papers supporting CBD in pain management, including the *Journal of Experimental Medicine*[viii] in 2012.

THC — Has psychoactive properties, but these are largely cancelled out when mixed with CBD. It's useful for epilepsy, works as an anti-inflammatory, protects the nervous system and works as a muscle relaxant

How psychoactive is THC?

It's the THC content that makes medical cannabis products containing it illegal in some countries. Forty-eight countries have embraced it though, making preparations containing THC available on prescription, or over the counter.

The effect on the brain is not directly related to the per cent content in any preparation. So unlike percentages found on the labels of alcoholic drinks — the higher the per cent the more potent the brew — a high THC percentage is no guarantee that a particular marijuana strain will be more potent. It depends on which other cannabinoids are present.

The figure you need to look for is the milligram content. Under 0.2mg, and you won't feel any effect. At 10mg, you will feel an effect but with a high level of CBD, the psychoactive effect will be much less, or negligible. THC, at say 20mg, has a clear psychoactive effect which suits some people but not others. Your senses become heightened, which can be helpful if you're suffering from cancer, multiple sclerosis, chronic fatigue syndrome or depression. The THC gives you a lift.

What can THC help?

- In 2009, scientists at the University of South Carolina, Columbia,[ix] found it worked as an anti-inflammatory agent and found that it has properties that can protect the nervous system from damage.

- Back in 1998, researchers from a medical lab in Maryland, US,[x] discovered it is also an antioxidant, a mechanism of protection of the nervous system.

- THC acts as a muscle relaxant and is given to multiple sclerosis patients who suffer stiff and painful muscles. It is used in Sativex, the first prescription medication derived from cannabis. (Sativex is one of the few cannabis derivatives that is licensed as a medicine in many countries. It contains around 50 per cent THC and 50 per cent CBD. The 50/50 split means that Sativex has no significant psychoactive affect as THC is nicely balanced out by CBD.)

- THC also acts as an appetite stimulant which is helpful for illnesses where weight loss is a problem.

- It is also used in epilepsy medicine and is particularly helpful for hard to treat childhood epilepsy.

CAUTION: Large amounts of THC, not balanced by CBD, can have a negative effect, causing anxiety and paranoia. These are transient feelings and will not cause permanent harm in the short term.

Minor Cannabinoids with Major Impact
Cannabinoids other than CBD and THC are known as minor cannabinoids, although this is is the wrong name as most of these minor cannabinoids are medicinal and can have a big impact. Here are the main four.

Cannabigerol (CBG) — is non-psychoactive and is anti-inflammatory, antibacterial and stimulates appetite
The cannabis plant contains less than 1 per cent of CBG. It's a big hitter though and is described as the stem-cell of cannabis — one of the first cannabinoids in the plant to develop — giving birth to all others.

In common with virtually all cannabinoids that have been studied so far, it does have medicinal properties:

- In animal models, Italian scientists from the University of Naples in 2013,[xi] found it had a positive effect on inflammatory bowel disease.
- Italian researchers in 2008, from the University of Eastern Piedmont, Novara, Italy,[xii] found it contains antibacterial properties.
- In 2015, at Complutense University in Madrid, Spain,[xiii] scientists found it helped animal models in Huntington's disease.
- A study in 2015, by researchers at the University of Naples, Italy,[xiv] discovered it had a positive effect on weak bladders. A year earlier in 2014,[xv] a different team at the same university found it stopped colon cancer cell growth
- At the University of Lodz in Poland in 2008,[xvi] researchers in the Visual Rehabilitation Clinic found that CBG may have a positive effect on glaucoma.

Cannabinol (CBN) — is slightly psychoactive and can help you sleep, is anti-convulsive, helps appetite, acts as a painkiller and stimulates bone growth after fractures

A little bit of CBN goes a long way.

- Japanese scientists from Hokuriku University, Kanazawa, Japan,[xvii] said as far back as 1995, that it can help you sleep and that it's as effective as a 10mg dose of the sleeping pill diazepam.
- The *Journal of Neuroscience*[xviii] reports it relieves pain.

- The *Journal of Neuroimmunology*[xix] suggests it is anti-inflammatory.
- Italian scientists from the University of Eastern Piedmont, Novara, Italy,[xx] say it is antibacterial.
- It has been shown to be anti-convulsive.
- It has also been shown to be able to stimulate appetite and promote the growth of bone after fractures.

Cannabichromene (CBC) — is non-psychoactive, can help brain stem cells regenerate, inhibits tumour growth, helps with pain, is antibacterial and stimulates bone growth

Discovered 50 years ago, CBC is prominent in medical research and its benefits look promising.

- In 2013, the Italian Endocannabinoid Research Group, from the Institute of Biomolecular Chemistry, Napoli, Italy,[xxi] suggested that CBC can help brain stem cells regenerate.
- They also suggest that it inhibits the growth of cancerous tumours. It interacts with a chemical we produce naturally called anandamide, which can fight breast cancer.
- Like other cannabinoids it helps with pain, is antibacterial and can stimulate bone growth which could help osteoporosis sufferers in the future.

Full extract oils and the entourage effect

Full extract medical cannabis oils — oils with a mix of cannabinoids and terpenes — are often more effective. The entourage effect describes the cannabis compounds working together. Sometimes pure THC or pure CBD (called isolates) medicines are not enough for some conditions. Whole plant medicine utilises all the cannabinoids which may be more beneficial.

Researchers, for example, in Canada have recently shown that full extract cannabis oil containing a mixture of cannabinoids, is at least as good and possibly better at controlling epilepsy in young children than the pure CBD-only medicine.

In other words, all the components of the plant probably act better together than the individual components alone.

Terpenes – such as alpha-pinene, myrcene, limonene, carophyllene, linalool

The cannabis plant also contains terpenes, essential oils that are responsible for how plants and flowers smell and give cannabis its characteristic aroma. Different terpenes give different aromas to different varieties of cannabis, in the same way they do to flowers, shrubs, fruit and vegetables.

There are, like the cannabinoids, well over 100 known terpenes in the plant world and over 100 are found in the cannabis plant. Not only do terpenes provide the smell but they also have medicinal properties.

Flavonoids — such as quercetin, beta-sitosterol, cannaflavin

Flavonoids are pigments that give flowers and other parts of plants their colour. They do more than make petals and leaves look pretty and scientists are now discovering they have their own medicinal properties. Research is in its early stages, but initial reports look encouraging.

Licensed synthetic medical cannabis developed by drugs companies

There are companies who have developed pure medicinal cannabis compounds like, for example, the 99.9 per cent pure CBD that was used in trials of the epilepsy drug called **Epidiolex**. Developed by the

18

British company G W Pharmaceuticals,[xxii] Epidiolex, is used to treat drug resistant childhood epilepsy and is the first pure CBD cannabis product to receive approval in any country and is now licensed in the USA.

Cannabis products developed by drug companies have generic and trade names – as do over-the-counter drugs. Ibuprofen is the generic name for Nurofen, for example. Nurofen is its trade name. In the list of prescription cannabis below, the generic name comes first, and the trade name is in brackets. For example: **nabiximols (Sativex)**.

- **cannabidiol (Epidiolex)** is 99 per cent pure CBD, 0.15 per cent THC and contains minor cannabinoids and other compounds. Used to treat drug resistant childhood epilepsy, it is the first pure CBD cannabis product to receive approval in any country.
  It is not currently available in the UK and Europe but should be sometime in 2019. It is available in the US

- **dronabinol (Marinol and Syndros)**, a synthetic THC, treats nausea and vomiting after chemotherapy, and anorexia in people suffering with AIDS.
  It is not currently available in the UK. It is available in the US

- **nabilone (Cesamet)** is a synthetic THC, also licensed to treat severe nausea and vomiting caused by chemotherapy treatment for cancer.
  It is available in the UK and has been available in the US since 1985

- **nabiximols (Sativex)** was licensed in 2010 and is a pure combination of 50 per cent CBD, and 50 per cent THC, prescribed to relieve multiple sclerosis spasticity symptoms.
  NICE has said that Sativex is not cost effective, although it is allowed in Wales who have a different NICE system and feel it is cost effective. It is not prescribed on the NHS by doctors outside Wales

and it is not available in Scotland or Northern Ireland. It is waiting for approval in the US.

- **Sativex** is sprayed under the tongue or inside the cheeks. It March 2019, it cost £375 for three vials, each containing 90 doses. The lowest daily dose is 4 sprays; the highest daily dose is 12 sprays. According to the MHRA, the daily cost of Sativex is between £5.56 - £16.68 per day

CHAPTER 2

Why our body works so well with medical cannabis

Our Endocannabinoid System (ECS)

This is an important part of the jigsaw and explains why medical cannabis works for so many conditions, but if you prefer, you can skip to chapter 3 to find out which health conditions medical cannabis can help.

Why should a plant have such a profound effect on our brain and other organs? It's only recently that we have been able to answer that question and it is because we have a human cannabinoid system that works with the cannabis plant. We have receptors that react specifically to cannabinoids in the cannabis plant. Those receptors are called cannabinoid type 1 (CB1) and cannabinoid type 2 (CB2).

This was only discovered in 1990, by Professor Raphael Mechoulam, an organic chemist from Israel who is considered the grandfather of medical cannabis. (He also identified CBD and THC). Scientists then found that ECS systems exist everywhere in our bodies: in our brain, liver, reproductive system, heart, bowel, bladder, gut and muscles.

Cannabinoids from the cannabis plant interact with our ECS system, a neurotransmitter system that communicates between our brain and body.

It seems that the ECS has a major role to play in many, if not all, bodily functions. So, it is not surprising that when we take cannabinoids from the cannabis plant, their interaction with our own endocannabinoid systems produces wide ranging effects (both positive and negative) on many different symptoms and diseases.

The endocannabinoid system is a neurotransmitter system

The ECS is a neurotransmitter system and there are many different neurotransmitter systems in our body, each controlling something different:

- The **dopamine system**: produces the feel-good hormone dopamine and sends chemical messages from the brain to the body. It is the system that malfunctions in Parkinson's disease
- The **noradrenaline system**: noradrenaline is a stress hormone that triggers our 'fight or flight' response
- The **GABAergic system**: gamma-aminobutyric acid (GABA) is mainly involved in inhibiting nerve impulses — moving the brain and body to a lower gear
- The **serotonin system**: the neurotransmitter serotonin helps regulate mood, social behaviour, appetite, digestion, sleep, memory, sexual desire and function

The ECS behaves slightly differently from other neurotransmitters. It turns off responses rather than on, and stops our body releasing chemicals that would over-stimulate our system. At least one role of the ECS is to keep us on an even keel. For example, it makes sure we're not too hot or cold.

Function of the Endocannabinoid System

The ECS has a role across the entire nervous system. Its key functions are:

Memory

It plays a significant role in memory. We know that smoking cannabis high in THC can impair short term memory. We know from animal models that the ECS is involved in learning. Much learning is carried out in part of the brain called the hippocampus, which is associated with memory. We know the ECS can facilitate growth of nerves in the hippocampus region in the adult brain. Maybe, in the future, we can manipulate the ECS to improve memory in people, for example, with dementia.

Pain Control

It is well known that the ECS plays a role in pain control. Cannabinoids suppress pain responses by adjusting the effects of other neurotransmitter systems, such as the noradrenaline system and the GABAergic system. The management of chronic pain is a key clinical role for cannabis.

Sleep

We know that our brain ECS is involved in promoting sleep and also has a role in the circadian rhythm, the body's system that promotes sleep and wakefulness over 24 hours.
A well-known effect of cannabis is that it can improve sleep and also cause daytime drowsiness. This doesn't have to be a negative effect, it can be calming, but the first time you try it, test it to see whether it might affect your reactions the following day. If it does, avoid driving or operating machinery.

Appetite

The ECS seems to have a key role in appetite stimulation. Mice that have deliberately had the CB1 receptor knocked out are less hungry and leaner than the mice that have the receptor. We know that cannabinoids can have a positive effect on appetite and we also know that some other cannabinoids can have the opposite effect and may have a role as anti-obesity agents.

Stress Response

The system has a role to play in the human stress response, although exactly what that role is, is still unclear.

Energy Balance and Metabolism

The balancing effect of the cannabinoids helps with the balance of the body's metabolic functions. The system also seems to have a role in adjusting sensitivity to insulin, which could make it important in controlling obesity and diabetes.

Anxiety and Social Behaviour

The endocannabinoid system also regulates anxiety behaviour, both in animals and in humans. Some neurotransmitter systems seem to promote an anxiety that in some circumstances can be useful, while the ECS seems to have the opposite effect. Again, the ECS provides checks and balances.

Immune Function

The CB1 receptor is mainly, but not exclusively, focused on the nervous system, whereas the CB2 receptor, is present in the nervous system, but found more widely outside the brain and spinal cord. CB2 has a particular role in the immune system. The ECS seems to have a protective role against inflammation, for example, it might play a role relieving symptoms, or at least slowing disease progression, in inflammatory conditions such as multiple sclerosis.

Runners' 'High' and Physical Exercise

The endocannabinoid anandamide, is a chemical found in the body which increases as a result of physical exercise. It is also associated with euphoria and mood lifting effects. This may explain the euphoria of the runners' 'high', as levels increase when you exercise. THC has a similar euphoric effect producing the high for recreational users.

Temperature Control

Anandamide and 2-AG (another endocannbinoid found in the body associated with pain relief) in animal models, have been shown to act on our temperature controlling systems.

CHAPTER 3

Which health conditions respond to medical cannabis?

Medical cannabis relieves symptoms

It doesn't matter what disease lies behind a particular symptom medical cannabis will help with the symptoms regardless.

Take pain for example. We know that cannabis is a pain reliever and fortunately it doesn't seem to matter whether the pain is caused by arthritis, cancer or nerve injury, cannabis will help.

We also know that cannabis is anti-epileptic and can reduce seizure numbers regardless of the underlying diagnosis that causes the seizures. So it doesn't matter whether the epilepsy is caused by a head injury, an infection such as meningitis, a vessel in the brain that hasn't formed properly, or a stroke, or whether it's simply the third of epilepsy sufferers who have no obvious cause for their seizures other than a low seizure threshold. All can benefit from medical cannabis.

What is the evidence that it works?

Medical cannabis is already legal in 48 of 195 countries, and, once more countries allow it for sale, further studies will be done, and the evidence will improve.

I have listed conditions under 'strong evidence', 'medium evidence' and 'less evidence'. If your particular symptom or condition is ranked as having less evidence, this does not mean cannabis will not work for that symptom or condition. It simply means that double-blind placebo-controlled trials (where neither the scientist nor the patient knows who is receiving the medical cannabis and who is receiving a placebo, so they can't be influenced), or the numbers of good quality studies available are fewer than with strong evidence.

For example, in pharmaceutical terms, the medical evidence for treating depression is 'less', but the reality is that many tens of thousands of people would not be using cannabis for depression if it did not help. There are very few studies that have shown conclusively that cannabis does help depression, but take John's story:

Case Study

John, age 48, suffered anxiety and depression for many years after his wife died. He struggled to cope alone, caring for his three children. His GP and psychiatrist prescribed antidepressants, but he didn't like the side effects which were mainly dry mouth, constipation and tiredness, as they interfered with his work at an engineering plant. He was so badly affected, he thought he might have to give up his job. At first, he smoked cannabis recreationally, just to numb his symptoms then switched to medical cannabis. The cannabis didn't just numb his symptoms it improved them and after 10 weeks, he successfully came off his antidepressants. He has not needed them for four years now. While he wouldn't claim to be one hundred per cent cured, he feels much better, is coping with his children, his job and his everyday life — and no debilitating side-effects.

Conditions where there is strong evidence

Anxiety, epilepsy, muscle spasm, nausea and vomiting after chemotherapy, pain.

Anxiety

There are few double blind placebo controlled studies in this area, however, two or three reviews, (including my own)[xxiii] concluded that there was strong evidence for the anti-anxiety effect of CBD. This is sometimes in combination with existing anti-anxiety drugs, or sometimes it can replace anti-anxiety medication (like the benzodiazepines lorazepam and diazepam for example).

In 2011, neuroscientists in Brazil[xxiv] tested medical cannabis on patients with a fear of public speaking and found that CBD significantly reduced their anxiety.

Remember, it is only CBD that helps anxiety. As a rough guide, start with 20mg to 30mg of CBD per day building up to about 100mg daily.

Epilepsy

Medicinal cannabis is particularly useful for drug-resistant childhood epilepsy.

Most of the evidence is with Dravet syndrome — an epilepsy syndrome that often features in people with autism, ADHD and with physical and learning delays — and Lennox-Gastaut Syndrome (LGS), characterised by multiple seizures and developmental delay. There is no reason why cannabis should not work in other epilepsy syndromes.

Epidiolex is licensed in the US for use with these syndromes. Some high-profile child cases have responded to CBD products, but have had an even better response with a very small amount of added THC.

How would you feel about giving medical cannabis to your child?

We need to take into account the effect of standard anti-convulsant drugs on children. These drugs come with significant side effects in terms of cognition and behaviour. When you consider there are over 90 known side-effects associated with anti-epilepsy drugs, like fatigue, tiredness, vomiting, weakness, dry mouth, dizziness, blood disorders, and serious problems like liver damage, if taking cannabis can reduce these drugs, this is clearly beneficial.

Case Study

A case that made headlines in the UK is the story of six-year-old Alfie Dingley. Diagnosed age four with a rare form of epilepsy that causes seizures and developmental delays, Alfie suffered up to 300 epileptic seizures a month and was hospitalised every 4 to 10 days. His doctors tried many anti-epilepsy drugs with no effect at all. Eventually, only steroids helped control his fits. His mother Hannah Deacon said: 'It's the most horrendous thing I've ever experienced. The steroids made him aggressive, he couldn't go to school. He would scratch, bite and punch me.'

In desperation, his family took him to Holland where doctors prescribed a high CBD, full extract, cannabis product. This helped him, but when 2mg of THC was added, his seizures dramatically improved. His parents then fought a brave campaign to get him a license so that the THC product could be imported into the UK. They succeeded, and Alfie is now on a high CBD product with a little THC; a combination that has fully controlled his seizures. His behaviour has improved and he is learning at school, as well as riding a bike and a horse. An astonishing improvement.

Dosage

Some children have taken really high doses of CBD, up to 1000mg or more of pure CBD Epidiolex daily. Remember that a dose of pure CBD in Epidiolex, is much higher than a dose of full extract CBD, so you may need about 200mg to 300mg of full extract CBD daily. If the response is good stick with it, but if not add a small amount of THC. Just 2mg to 3mg daily, can produce a dramatic improvement.

Many people worry about the psychoactive effect of THC in children, but a very small dose of THC combined with a high dose of CBD means that the combined effect is not psychoactive. CBD easily counteracts the THC effect.

Most children with epilepsy have tried several different standard anti-convulsant drugs before trying cannabis. Some can come off all their other standard anti-epilepsy drugs. The majority still need one, or a few, of the standard anticonvulsants in addition to the cannabis products.

As there is an element of trial and error, supervision by an expert paediatrician or paediatric neurologist is advised, often with the input and help of a cannabis physician if you have access to one. In the UK, there are only a few doctors who know how to prescribe cannabis but that should change in 2019. Three private medical cannabis clinics plan to open in the Spring/Summer of 2019 in London, Manchester and Birmingham. The NHS should follow.

In Canada, where cannabis is fully legal, it's sold openly in shops and the 'budtenders' are like pharmacists, extremely knowledgeable when it comes to prescribing the right medical cannabis. Most take courses in how to prescribe, but there is no university degree as yet.

Family doctors can also refer patients to cannabis specialists like the Canadian website cannabisclinics.ca.

In the 33 states where medical cannabis is legal in the US, high street stores with budtenders sell medical cannabis, like in Canada. It is also available on prescription and the Marijuana Doctors website can recommend good doctors in each state.

Muscle Spasm
Case Study
Age 28, Gillian was diagnosed with multiple sclerosis. First her hand co-ordination and speech deteriorated, then she began having problems walking because of muscle spasms. Confined to a wheelchair, she tried three drugs to help with this, (baclofen, dantrium and gabapentin), without much effect. Her doctor suggested Sativex and after a few weeks, her spasms improved, and she was able to control her legs better. She still takes baclofen but supplements it with sprays of Sativex when she knows she will need more control. For example, like going out in the evening when she may be getting in and out of a car.

The evidence that medical cannabis helps relax muscle spasms is good. Most trials are with multiple sclerosis patients, but this does not mean that cannabis will not work for the other causes of muscle spasm, such as brain injury, stroke, spinal injury and motor neurone disease.

The most commonly used medical cannabis as a muscle relaxant is Sativex — 50 per cent THC and 50 per cent CBD in pure form, available as a spray under the tongue. Both CBD and THC have anti-spasm effects. So, if Sativex is not available then there is no right or wrong alternative. It is best, at first, to try a strain high in CBD and low in THC, to minimise any psychoactive side effects.

Nausea and Vomiting after Chemotherapy

Nausea and sickness in chemotherapy can be debilitating, but as Dame Sally Davies' review[xxv] confirms, cannabis is helpful controlling nausea and vomiting associated with chemotherapy during cancer treatment. Synthetic nabilone and dronabinol are licensed as treatments but are not that different to standard prescription drugs.

The THC component here is usually more important than the CBD component. It is worth trying a balanced CBD/THC product first before increasing the THC. It is also initially worth trying more standard anti-sickness drugs (like metoclopramide and prochlorperazine), and if the effect is poor, then add a cannabis product.

CAUTION: Medical cannabis is not recommended for nausea and vomiting caused by pregnancy.

Pain

One of the most comprehensive reviews produced in 2017, by the National Academies of Sciences, Engineering and Medicine in the US[xxvi] (a private, nonprofit institution providing expert advice on science, engineering and medicine to governments and other organisations) says that there is conclusive evidence that cannabis is effective for the treatment of chronic pain in adults. As chronic pain affects more people than cancer, diabetes and heart disease combined, and is the most common cause of disability, this is good news for pain sufferers.

Evidence

According to a 2018 study by scientists from McGill University Medical School in Montreal, Canada,[xxvii] medical cannabis works for any type of pain. This includes pain from cancer, headache, arthritis or joint problems and nerve problems.

There are many more studies of different aspects of pain using the synthetic cannabinoids — nabilone, dronabinol — and Sativex, as well as studies using natural cannabis. We also know, both from animal models and human studies, that both CBD and THC are painkillers.

The Royal Orthopaedic Hospital in Middlesex, UK, conducted a trial into pain from shoulder and arm injury, using a 50/50 ratio of CBD and THC, and found that patients' sleep and pain improved, and any side-effects suffered were minimal and resolved by themselves.

'Opioid sparing'

Cannabis products are "opioid sparing", meaning that if you are taking opioid drugs for pain, such as morphine, fentanyl, codeine or methadone, if you take cannabis you can usually reduce the opioid dosage and sometimes even stop them altogether.

We've said this before but it's worth repeating. In states in the USA where medical cannabis has been introduced, there is around a 25 per cent reduction of opioid prescriptions. This is a significant breakthrough as deaths from opioid overdose, both accidental and deliberate, are a real problem around the world.

Deaths from prescription opioids in the US are around 49,000 a year, and 4,500 in the UK. *The introduction of cannabis could save 25 per cent of those deaths* and more if people were able to come off their opioid medication altogether. No one has ever died from a cannabis overdose.

What should I take?
The safest way to find out what works best for your pain is to start with a CBD full extract product, or with other minor cannabinoids and terpenes and not just CBD, and then add in THC gradually. Some online suppliers outside the UK have help and chat lines who can advise. (Go to page 113 for supplier details.)

Medical cannabis is very subtle, and each patient is different so slight tweaks in the CBD/THC ratio may make a difference. As THC is the element with the most side-effects, a good policy is to increase the THC dose gradually over time.

Dosage required?
CBD dosages would start quite low at between 20mg and 30mg daily building up to 100mg to 200mg daily, or more. Pure CBD (such as Epidiolex) will need higher dosing than full extract CBD containing other minor cannabinoids and terpenes.

With THC products, start low, at 1mg to 2mg daily, and build up to about 20mg or so daily.

Some people are very sensitive to cannabis dosing and require a very low dose — micro-dose — whilst others seem to be quite resistant and require higher doses. There is no right dose, it is a matter of starting at a low dose and slowly working up until you get the benefit, and carefully monitoring any unwanted side effects.

Conditions where there is medium evidence

Appetite stimulation, fibromyalgia, post-traumatic stress disorder (PTSD), sleep disorders

Appetite Stimulation

The journal *Nature Neuroscience,* published a study in 2014,[xxviii] by a team of European scientists from France, into how cannabis affects appetite. It showed that THC tricked the brain into thinking it was hungry.

There is a paradox here: While it helped people with low weight, gain weight, it didn't increase the weight of people who were normal weight or overweight. In a 2014 study conducted by Wright State University School of Medicine, Ohio, US,[xxix] into cannabis and body weight, they hypothesised that cannabis regulated the metabolism in people with low-weight but did not affect people who were normal-weight or overweight.

The 'munchies' is a well-known side effect of cannabis, and there is no doubt that the ECS plays a role in appetite. Poor appetite and weight loss can be a feature of debilitating diseases, such as HIV/Aids, or cancer. The THC component seems to improve appetite so maybe a 50/50 THC to CBD product is best at first before trying a higher THC strain.

Fibromyalgia

Fibromyalgia is a painful disorder of the central nervous system. Sufferers describe this condition, which affects the muscles, as a deep muscular aching, throbbing, shooting, stabbing or intense burning pain.

It's a common condition thought to effect 1 in 25, and more women than men, but responds well to medical cannabis.

A high CBD product is recommended starting with a low dose and building up. If there is limited effect with CBD, add a small amount of THC before moving to a higher THC product if it feels necessary

Case study
Anne, aged 42, has had fibromyalgia, in association with osteoarthritis for about 10 years. She needed opioids and other painkillers (including Naprosyn, a non-steroidal anti-inflammatory drug). Her sleep was poor, but mainly her life was miserable because of constant pain, mainly in her legs and shoulders. Reluctantly, she used a CBD product with some benefit estimating a 30 per cent to 40 per cent improvement. She then added a product with some THC (about 80:20 CBD to THC ratio) and the benefit was nearer 90 per cent. She still has painful days, but her pain is much less intrusive; and she is back at work. She had been signed off sick for 2 years beforehand. She even has a social life!

Case Study
Catherine, 68, from Britain, has been able to stop taking her opioids thanks to medical cannabis. She has suffered with fibromyalgia and arthritis for 20 years. To deal with excruciating pain, she was prescribed opioids, (like the powerful prescription painkiller and tranquilliser fentanyl, and the painkiller tramadol.) They all came with side effects like drowsiness, severe constipation and itching, and didn't help much. She also tried the anti-inflammatory drugs, aspirin and paracetamol, but nothing worked. Her sleep pattern was disturbed, and she suffered constant pain. Reluctant to try CBD, even though her husband was a qualified doctor, she came to the conclusion she had nothing to lose and took a full extract CBD capsule. It contained mainly CBD but other

minor cannabinoids, like CBDA, CBN, CBC and CBG. (More about these to follow.) Her brand was made by the Dutch company Endoca. She slowly built her daily dose up over two months from 20mg to 250mg. Slowly but surely, her pain lessened, and her sleep improved. She no longer needs her opioids, only occasionally taking the anti-inflammatory drug naprosyn when she has a particularly bad flare up.

Post-Traumatic Stress Disorder (PTSD)
Case Study

Derick was a soldier sent to the Falklands Islands, when Britain went to war with the Argentines over sovereignty in the early 1980s. He was in the thick of one of the main battles and witnessed some shocking scenes. He came home, left the armed forces and had huge trouble settling back into civilian life. He tried jobs in the police force, fire service and then sadly drifted into petty crime. He could not sleep, had flashbacks about the Falklands, got very anxious when he was in groups of people, and had panic attacks if he heard loud, unexpected noises. He began to drink excessively and was eventually diagnosed with post-traumatic stress disorder (PTSD). He was referred to a counselling service but did not go. A friend persuaded him to try smoking a joint, and after just one experience, he felt a little better that day. He didn't like smoking and was introduced to vaping, and oils for oral use. He has now found a balance between a regular oil (about 50 mg CBD) and an extra vape when he is going out in groups. He has found a job that he can manage as a night security guard at a supermarket. He is not cured and still gets anxious but is coping with life, has a job and has stopped drinking.

- In 2018, researchers from the Universities of South Santa Catarina and Santa Catarina in Brazil,[xxx] found good evidence that many people like Derick with PTSD, use cannabis to regulate their

37

symptoms to good effect. While in 2017, researchers at Oregon Health and Science University, and the Veterans Affairs Health Care System in Portland, Oregon, US,[xxxi] felt that there was not enough evidence.

- It is worth starting with a high CBD product as anxiety is usually a dominant feature in PTSD, before moving on, if need be, to more balanced strains.

Sleep Disorders

As many as 16 million UK adults, and up to 70 million adults in the US, suffer with sleep problems; almost 30 per cent in both populations. Many trials show that medical cannabis helps with sleep problems. A review of sleep studies in 2017, by researchers at Palo Alto University, California, US,[xxxii] showed a positive response with an improved overnight sleep pattern in 50 per cent of people using cannabis in various formats.

There are many causes for sleep disturbance all of which can be helped by medical cannabis:

- chronic pain
- anxiety
- muscle spasm
- restless leg syndrome

Case Study

Jane, 63, suffers chronic osteoarthritis, a condition where the protective cartilage at the ends of your bones breaks down, causing pain, swelling and problems moving the joint. For many years, she has found sleep difficult, often disturbed by her pain and by the fact that she cannot find a comfortable position in bed. To relieve her symptoms, she tried sleeping pills with no effect. They left her groggy the next morning and she hated the effect. Eventually, a friend persuaded her to try medical cannabis. She took full extract CBD obtained online from the Dutch company Endoca. She takes 300mg daily. Her pain and sleep have improved, and she now takes no other medication.

Which medical cannabis to use for sleep disturbance?

Products developed by drugs companies

The natural preparation nabiximols (Sativex) can help, and other studies have shown that synthetic nabilone (Cesamet), can be useful. In places where these drugs are not available in the UK with an NHS prescription, a doctor can give you a private prescription.

Natural product

In terms of the natural product, we know that sleep can be helped particularly, but by no means exclusively, by the indica strains. Choosing the right strain can be trial and error, a bit like choosing the right tea; should it be white or black, caffeinated or herbal? As a very general guide, indica is thought of as more soothing and relaxing while sativa strains are more likely to make you feel energised and happy. Then there are the hybrids, ask your manufacturer, dispensary or doctor to advise on hybrids, which are a mix of two strains.

Too much THC can make you feel groggy and sleepy in the morning, but on the other hand some find that higher THC varieties improves sleep. Cannabis may help you to fall asleep faster too. Some people notice they dream less. Cannabis that has aged slightly has a higher CBN content. Some find this is better for sleep, although the theory has not yet been put through formal tests.

Taking capsules or edibles will last through the night while vaping or taking drops tends to have a shorter-term effect. For those new to vaping, a vape machine works like an electronic cigarette — it heats the cannabis oil or tincture until it vaporises, you then inhale the vapour. Bear in mind that edibles can take between one to three hours to take effect. Taking your required dose an hour before you want to sleep is recommended.

Conditions where there is less evidence

There is some evidence that medical cannabis works for the following, but it's not a huge volume. This doesn't mean that it doesn't work, or that it is not worth trying, just that we need more studies to confirm the results.

Alzheimer's disease and dementia, amyotrophic lateral sclerosis (ALS) and motor neurone disease (MND), attention deficit hyperactivity disorder (ADHD) and attention deficit disorder (ADD), autistic spectrum disorders, bladder problems, bowel problems, brain injury, cancer, depression, eye symptoms, headache and migraine, Huntington's disease, obsessive compulsive disorder (OCD), Parkinson's disease, psychosis, spinal cord injury, Tourette's syndrome

Alzheimer's disease and dementia

Globally, almost 50 million people suffer with Alzheimer's and dementia; 5.7 million are in the US, while 850,000 are in the UK. By 2025, these figures are set to increase by almost 15 per cent.

A team from the independent medical research unit Neuroscience Research Australia,[xxxiii] studied mice with Alzheimer's symptoms and found in 2017, that a combination of THC and CBD, dramatically improved their memory. They discovered it affected the way a destructive protein called amyloid develops. Amyloid can cluster and form tangles inside neurons (nerve cells) in dementia patients, causing the classic symptoms of memory loss, problems communicating, concentrating, reasoning, and judgement.

Also, in dementia, and particularly in Alzheimer's, there is an enzyme (acetylcholinesterase) that if inhibited seems to slow the progression of Alzheimer's disease. From early studies conducted by the Skaggs Institute for Chemical Biology, California, US, in 2006,[xxxiv] we know that THC can inhibit that enzyme.

Cannabis products can help with anxiety and agitation. Anecdotal reports say that CBD can help the anxiety associated with early stage dementia. There is a 2018 study from Sunnybrook Health Sciences Centre, University of Toronto, Canada[xxxv] that has shown a positive effect on agitation caused by dementia using the synthetic THC nabilone.

For six weeks, they gave the pill to 39 patients with dementia, then gave them a placebo for six more weeks. The Alzheimer's Association in the US said: "Agitation improved significantly in those taking nabilone, compared to placebo. Nabilone also significantly improved overall behavioural symptoms, compared to placebo, as measured by the Neuropsychiatric Inventory questionnaire."

Amyotrophic Lateral Sclerosis (ALS), also known as Motor Neurone Disease (MND)
There are two names for this condition:
- Amyotrophic lateral sclerosis (ALS), which is mainly used in the US

41

- Motor neurone disease (MND), which is mainly used in the UK and Europe
- It is also known as Lou Gehrig's disease in the US

Motor neurone disease is a rare, degenerative, neurological disease involving the nerve cells controlling voluntary muscle movement. The average person with MND/ALS will live for two years after diagnosis. They are troubled by muscle spasm as well as, in the later stages, by anorexia, weight loss and the need for appetite stimulation. Cannabis can be useful to help some of those symptoms.

Case study

One case study, published in 2017 in the *Journal of General Practice*,[xxxvi] described how an Austrian MND patient, suffering weakness in his leg, foot, hand and tongue, was prescribed a drug (riluzole) to slow down his symptoms. After eight weeks, there was no change and his MND was progressing relatively quickly. He decided to try 2 x 200mg of CBD daily with his riluzole. He then increased his CBD to 2 x 300mg daily. Within six weeks, the weakness in his hand and foot had reversed completely. His tongue improved a little but deteriorated again after 10 weeks. He lost his speech after 18 months, but his limbs were much slower to deteriorate.

In other words, in his case, the cannabis may have slowed down the disease.

Autistic spectrum disorders (ASDs)

Evidence is emerging that cannabis can help people with autism.

Autism is a spectrum of disorders that impact on development of the brain, often characterised by communication problems, difficulties with social interaction and repetitive and difficult behaviours like self-

42

harming, as well as aggressive behaviour like biting, spitting and hair pulling.

There are no clinical studies for medical cannabis and autism but there is a growing body of positive anecdotal evidence. Some of the drugs used to treat autism, (like the antipsychotics risperidone and aripiprazole), are said to help with aggression but can be associated with significant side effects like weight gain, restlessness, tremors and tics.

There is some evidence that the ECS can be involved in autism. Italian scientists looked at the role of the ECS in ASDs and found that it was affected in patients with ASD diagnoses.

Bladder Problems
There are cannabinoid receptors in the bladder.

Trials, sponsored by G W Pharmaceuticals, prescribing Sativex for people with MS who suffer with two types of bladder problem — frequent urination, or problems urinating — show that episodes of incontinence at night, and the number of trips to the bathroom during the day, improved. But in fairness, other studies have failed to show any improvement.

Bowel Problems
Many people take cannabis for gastrointestinal problems like Crohn's disease, ulcerative colitis and irritable bowel syndrome (IBS). There are many positive stories of the benefits of cannabis products, particularly for Crohn's disease and IBS.

Case study

Take Juliette for example, who has a long history of Crohn's disease dating back 10 years. She suffers with severe diarrhoea with abdominal pains. She also gets very tired and struggles to maintain a reasonable weight, which she loses easily.

She tried most known drugs that help Crohn's including steroids, (such as sulphasalazine, and methotrexate), antibiotics and standard painkillers, as well as anti-diarrhoea drugs. The only thing that had helped to some extent were steroids.

She tried a medical cannabis vape and used a high THC product. It has helped her a little and she has managed to reduce her steroid dose. The diarrhoea continues but is less frequent and with less pain. She is also sleeping better, and her appetite has improved. She is not cured but the medical cannabis has improved her quality of life.

Other case studies

- Many case study audits have shown significant use of medical cannabis amongst people with similar problems, which should imply that it is helpful for some people.

- The gastrointestinal system hosts CB1 and CB2 receptors and activating these receptors improves bowel movements, as well as production of gastric juices and stomach emptying. In some circumstances, cannabis can be anti-inflammatory so is helpful with conditions that are characterised by inflammation, like Crohn's disease and ulcerative colitis.

- Medical cannabis can reduce muscle spasm making it helpful for IBS.

- It is worth trying a balanced CBD:THC product first, before moving towards a higher THC product.

Brain Injury
Case study

Lewis was 24 when he was run over at a pedestrian crossing. The car was driven by a drunk driver. He was immediately transferred to a neurosurgical centre to have a blood clot on his brain removed, but this left him with brain damage on the right side of his brain. He was discharged from hospital after three months, having made some recovery, although he still suffered severe and painful muscle spasms in his left arm and leg, which stopped him doing simple tasks like dressing himself.

The change in his life began to get him down and he became anxious. His sleep was affected, and he began to neglect himself. He lost his job and his girlfriend left him. His consultant prescribed drugs for his spasms (baclofen) and for his sleep (benzodiazepines). The only thing that made a real difference was counselling. His counsellor suggested trying cannabis.

Lewis was reluctant but obtained some recreational oil from a friend who showed him how to vape it. (See chapter 4 on how to take medical cannabis.) He also began to try cannabis edibles, working out the best dose and strain for himself. After several months of trial and error, he found a balance between eating cannabis brownies twice a day, and vaping in the morning and evening, and an extra vape at midday if he was home at lunch time. He got most benefit from high CBD cannabis, with around 300mg CBD and about 5mg THC. The result for Lewis is less muscle spasms, less pain, better appetite and better sleep. The next step for him is to get back to work, but in the meantime, he is managing to live alone and is managing his life.

- Traumatic brain injury symptoms can include, pain, anxiety, headache, memory loss and depression
- In 2014, a small study by researchers at Harbor-UCLA Medical Centre in Torrance, California, US,[xxxvii] found that the survival rate amongst the 18 per cent of brain injury, or brain haemorrhage patients, who had taken cannabis at some point in the previous weeks and tested positive for THC in toxicology tests, was significantly higher. Only two died in the THC positive group, while 42 died in the group that tested negative for THC. In this study it seems that THC had a protective effect
- A concussion pill is being developed by The University of Miami Miller School of Medicine and The Miami Project to Cure Paralysis, both in California, US, and Sol Global Investments Corp in Toronto, Canada.[xxxviii] "The results were statistically significant and encouraging," Scythian's Jonathan Gilbert, who manages the University of Miami partnership, said in 2018. "This evidence strongly suggests further testing is warranted on medical cannabis' potential in the treatment of trauma to the brain."

Cancer

In the US, almost 2 million people were diagnosed with cancer in 2018 and 600,000 died from the disease. In the UK, 360,000 are diagnosed annually and there are 164,000 deaths. The American Cancer Society[xxxix] says that men have a 1 in 3 risk of developing cancer, while for women, the odds are slightly lower. According to the British charity, Cancer Research,[xl] there is a 1 in 2 risk of developing cancer if you live in the UK.

- Cancer is the most destructive disease we face today with wildly different survival rates for the different types of cancer. According to Cancer Research UK, there is a 98 per cent survival rate[xli] from testicular cancer, which drops to just 1 per cent for pancreatic cancer. Cancer treatment with chemotherapy and radiotherapy is harsh, and common side-effects include hair loss, nausea, anaemia and fatigue

- Anything that can help with symptoms from treatment, as well as cancer symptoms, is welcome and medical cannabis is building a solid reputation in these areas. It can help with many cancer symptoms such as pain, nausea, muscle spasm, anxiety, appetite and sleep, while the quality of life for patients having cancer treatment is undoubtedly improved

- Dr. Wai Liu, a research fellow at St Georges University of London, UK, develops novel approaches to cancer treatment. He says of medical cannabis as a treatment for cancer: "Mechanistically, both THC and cannabinoids work by switching on cell killing processes that are found in cancer cells. Switching these on leads to cell death, reducing tumours. These signalling cascades could actually make the cancer cells more sensitive to other forms of therapy too."

- Cancer Research UK, fund clinical trials into medical cannabis as a cancer treatment. Dr. Kat Arney, said when she was science communications manager for Cancer Research UK: "We know that cannabinoids can have a range of different effects on cancer cells grown in the lab and animal tumours."

- Some of the most dramatic anecdotal tales of the effectiveness of medical cannabis are with cancer cures

Which cancers?

- It is very unlikely that cannabis can help all cancers as there are so many different types, with so many different causes, but one of the earliest papers, published in 1975 in the *Journal of the National Cancer Institute*,[xlii] showed that THC, and other cannabinoids, stopped tumour growth in lung cancer patients

- In 2005, researchers at the University of Wisconsin, US,[xliii] suggested that cannabis sativa could be used to treat prostate cancer

- Scientists at the University of Otago in New Zealand[xliv] used cannabis sativa to treat oestrogen receptive breast cancer in 2009

- There is certainly good quality evidence in animals that different cannabinoids, and some of the terpenes, have anti-cancer effects. In 2014, scientists from the Central Drug Research Institute in Lucknow, India and from the Department of Pathology at Ohio State University, Columbus, Ohio, US,[xlv] published a study that found that the cannabis sativa plant was effective in fighting cancer

Breast cancer, cancerous brain tumours and bladder cancer

- Patients report that medical cannabis works well with breast cancer, brain tumours and bladder cancer. There is some research in this area, but more is needed to get a stronger picture of the capabilities of medical cannabis

- There are three studies that provide some hope for patients suffering with aggressive brain cancer (gliobastoma multiforme)

- In 2017, G W Pharma carried out a placebo-controlled trial with 21 patients suffering with brain cancer (gliobastoma multiforme),[xlvi] which does not respond well to conventional treatments. They found by using chemotherapy, with THC and CBD, patients had an 83 per cent survival rate, compared with a 53 per cent survival rate for those using chemotherapy alone

- In 2014, St George's Hospital's oncology team, in London, UK,[xlvii] treated mice with malignant cancer tumours (gliomas) with radiotherapy, CBD and THC. They found that medical cannabis stopped the tumour growth and helped the anticancer effects of the radiation

- In 2011, using another mouse model, Complutense University in Madrid, Spain,[xlviii] who are advanced researchers into medical cannabis, found that THC and CBD, combined with chemotherapy, stopped brain cancer (gliobastoma multiforme) tumour growth. The treatment also helped clear out damaged cells and regenerate new ones. Researchers said: "We found this treatment has a strong, anti-tumour action."

- There are many anecdotal stories of people being cured of cancer by using cannabis, or at least having their survival prolonged. Here are three:

Case study

Luzita Hill, 52, from Britain, was diagnosed with oestrogen responsive breast cancer (ER-positive) in 2012. She had two lumpectomies, chemotherapy and daily radiotherapy and was clear for three years until 2016. As so often happens, her cancer came back and was found in her lungs and bones. Doctors said there was nothing they could do and gave her six months to live. She resigned herself to making the best of the time she had left, but a gift from a friend changed her life.

Luzita said: "I was given a pot of cannabis coconut oil by an herbalist friend. I rubbed it on an inoperable tumour on my shoulder and it disappeared." After that, Luzita began studying as a herbalist and made her own tincture with the whole plant. She began a medical cannabis

49

regime, is still alive and still applies a topical oil to her breast and shoulder area, made from whole plant extracts, takes a tincture daily, as well as eating and vaping the homegrown raw plant.

She said: "All my medical team know about my cannabis regime and they are happy for me to continue. I also have regular scans and 3-monthly oncology appointments."

Case study

Phil James, 32, is an academic from Wales who was diagnosed with a brain tumour in 2015. Doctors found a rare cancerous tumour (anaplastic astrocytoma) in his brain, after he suffered a seizure. The one-year survival rate for sufferers of this cancer is just over 50 per cent, dropping to 30 per cent for three years and under 20 per cent for five years.

In January 2016, he had surgery to remove 80 per cent of his tumour. This was followed by radiotherapy to slow down the tumour growth. Doctors expected his tumours to grow back slowly and were simply buying him time.

That same year, Phil began taking a CBD tincture made by a US company called Charlotte's Web available from Savage Cabbage in the UK. He also placed a CBD patch on his foot before bed and also vaped the cannabis plant to take advantage of the entourage effect. He changed to a Ketogenic diet, which is no sugar, high in fat and low in carbohydrate After four years, he has remained seizure free and eight brain scans have shown only a minimal trace of his tumour.

He said: "I was told I had two years to live. I was told there was nothing that could be done. I took advice about using cannabidiol from St George's University[xlix] in London, UK, who wrote a paper showing the effects of CBD indica on glioma (brain cancer). I also changed to a strict, healthy diet. I put my survival down to diet and taking CBD."

Case Study

Trevor Smith, 59, from the UK was diagnosed with bladder cancer in 2012. He was given 18-months to live by two top urologists unless he had radical surgery to remove not only his bladder, prostate and lymph nodes, but some intestines to re-build a new bladder. Trevor's doctors urged him to have surgery immediately, and to also have chemotherapy and radiotherapy. He decided he would rather take the 18-months of life as he was a manager in the oil and gas industry, and such radical surgery would have changed his quality of life hugely.

His wife Carol, 59, then began looking for alternative solutions. She changed his diet cutting out red meat, processed foods, dairy products and sugar. Trevor took alternative medicines such as Essiac tea, an herbal tea that is said to help cure cancer, green detox powders and food supplements. He visited alternative doctors and had blood tests that proved he was deficient in vitamins C and D; so, he took high doses of both. He also took vitamin K and B17 and the hormone dehydroepiandrosterone (DHEA), which is naturally produced by the body and boosts immune function.

Then, 9 months after he began this journey of healing, Carol read about medical cannabis, and although it wasn't legal in the UK then, Carol and Trevor both decided it was worth the risk and added it to his protocol. The father of three, took 60gm of 65 per cent THC medical cannabis oil over a period of 10 weeks. He suffered side effects from the medical cannabis, feeling sleepy and unresponsive at times, but persisted. After 10 weeks, doctors said that although his tumours had increased they were still in his bladder and hadn't metastasized and spread to his other organs, which meant they could remove them with conventional laser therapy. The laser therapy worked, the tumours were completely removed and Trevor avoided radical surgery, chemotherapy and radiotherapy.

His wife Carol says: "Trevor did many things, but I believe that medical cannabis stopped the metastasis so that Trevor's tumours were contained in his bladder. After the laser treatment, Trevor had a BCG (a type of immunotherapy vaccine) into his bladder and he stayed cancer free for four and a half years."

A superficial tumour was then found and was lasered and he had another BCG. This has happened twice since then, but Trevor is still cancer free.

Carol said: "It has been over seven years since doctors gave him 18-months to live. He does not regret trying alternative therapies, including medical cannabis."

Depression

- According to the World Health Organisation,[l] 350 million people worldwide suffer with depression and annually there are 800,000 suicides related to depression

- Cannabis use for depression is really common and has been used for centuries. Scientists are now discovering why: medical cannabis seems to realign the ECS which becomes unbalanced in depression and pain

- According to a 2018 survey by the United Patients Alliance (UPA),[li] a British support group for patients using cannabis, 17 per cent of patients say they use street cannabis for depression making it the second commonest reason for cannabis use after pain

- Depression often goes hand in hand with anxiety, which may explain why it helps with depression. There is a great deal of anecdotal and case study evidence that cannabis formulations can be used for depression, but few trials have been done

Eye Symptoms

Cannabis can help the symptoms of glaucoma which is the second leading cause of blindness in the world. It is characterised by increased pressure of fluid on the optic nerve inside the eye.

The ECS is present throughout the eye tissues and pressure from fluid can be lowered by using cannabinoids. In 2016, Canadian researchers from Dalhousie University, Halifax,[lii] showed that a small dose of THC, of around 5mg, reduced pressure, but CBD did not.

There are too few good quality studies available to come to a conclusive conclusion, but early reports look promising.

Headache and Migraine

For centuries, cannabis has been used to treat migraine or headache and it's one of the earliest described uses of the plant.

- The American psychopharmacology researcher and pioneer in cannabis science Ethan Russo, suggested in a paper published in 2004 in the international journal *Neuroendocrinology Letters,*[liii] that there is an: 'endocannabinoid deficiency syndrome'. He believes this might explain the underlying cause of many immune system disorders. His theory is that the body doesn't produce enough endocannabinoids or enough receptors for the system to function properly

- Examining the literature, he found that some people had lower levels of endocannabinoids and/or cannabinoid receptors and that these people were susceptible to conditions like migraine, fibromyalgia and irritable bowel syndrome. This might explain why cannabis seems to work so well for these conditions

- Because cannabis has been used for so many years to treat headache and migraine, there are few scientific studies looking into it.

- Conventional treatments can be hit and miss and triptans, which are commonly prescribed for migraines, come with side-effects like drowsiness, dizziness, nausea, tingling or numbness in the toes, or tightness in the chest or throat

Case study

Roseanne, now 32, has had migraine since she was a young girl. She suffered really badly at the time of her periods. She tried everything she could to alleviate the problem and had been prescribed all the standard medicines, including triptans, simple analgesics with anti-nausea medication, beta blockers and anti-depressants. She had also tried over the counter preparations such as Migraleve. She recently tried vaping a balanced THC and CBD product on advice from a friend, and found it helped the migraine once it started and made it last a shorter time. Vaping daily in the evening also seems to have reduced the frequency of the migraines, although it is early days.

Huntington's Disease

Huntington's disease is an inherited disorder resulting in brain cell death. Early symptoms include a lack of coordination and an unsteady walk, and problems with mood. Mental abilities are affected and can decline into dementia.

A small study of the synthetic cannabis nabilone, showed some improvement in comparison to placebo for motor problems and cognition, and some aspects of behaviour.

Obsessive Compulsive Disorder (OCD)

OCD is an anxiety disorder with two main symptoms, psychological and physical: obsessions and compulsions.

Around half of people who do not respond to standard medical treatment, such as antidepressants, cognitive behavioural therapy (CBT) and exposure therapy (which entails facing the fears that most haunt you) use cannabis. The anti-anxiety properties of CBD are what people find helpful although paradoxically, some find that THC can be useful.

Parkinson's Disease

- Parkinson's disease affects about 1 in every 350 people and is more common in men than women. It's a progressive nervous system disease that causes tremors in the limbs, mainly in the elderly.

- We know that stimulating the CB1 receptor can stimulate the dopamine system, which is the system depleted and the one mainly affected in Parkinson's.

- A 2014, double-blind placebo-controlled study by researchers from the University of São Paulo, Brazil,[liv] found that CBD helped improve Parkinson's symptoms like memory, mood, fatigue and weight. The same study saw an improvement in sufferers' tremors and another study from the University of São Paulo in 2018,[lv] showed some benefit from CBD (300mg) on well-being and quality of life with sufferers experiencing less stiffness, less anxiety and less pain. It also has positive effects on pain, anxiety and sleep.

Psychosis

Psychosis sufferers perceive and interpret things differently to others, they might also suffer hallucinations or delusions. High concentrations of THC, or THC in isolation, can trigger schizophrenia and/or psychotic episodes in susceptible people. A 2018 study from the University of Milan, Italy,[lvi] shows that CBD, with its calming effect, can be helpful as an anti-psychotic. It certainly has fewer side effects than some of the standard anti-psychotic drugs.

Spinal Cord Injury
- Muscle spasm is common in spinal cord injury if the part of the brain controlling movement is damaged. It can be a real issue, often painful and disabling
- Sativex is licensed for muscle spasm in MS so it is worth a trying it for muscle spasms caused by spinal cord injury
- Pain can also be a problem, especially nerve pain, and that can cause sleep problems. Those symptoms can be helped by cannabis, as we have seen

Tourette's syndrome
Tourette's syndrome is a neurological disorder characterised by involuntary tics and a compulsion to swear.

Two small studies from 2017, both from Hannover Medical School, Germany,[lvii] with THC showed some improvement with tics but not swearing. Patients were taking up to 10mg of THC daily. There are also anecdotal reports confirming usefulness.

Other symptoms and diseases
There are a number of other case reports and anecdotes showing some benefit in other conditions. The evidence is sparse for these conditions and mainly relies on case studies or small trials. I haven't gone into

extensive detail, but they are worth mentioning as the reports may point the way to future research.

Asthma — a serious condition in the lungs that causes difficulty in breathing

Hiccups

Isaac's syndrome — a rare condition associated with immune system dysfunction, that causes muscles to quiver

Night sweats — caused by the menopause and other issues

Night vision problems

Pruritus — itchy skin

Tinnitus — constant buzzing or ringing in one or both ears

Trichotillomania — compulsive hair pulling, including eyebrows and eyelashes

Cannabis treatment is approved in the US for other conditions
In the US, cannabis prescriptions for the following conditions and illnesses are approved in some, or all, of 38 states:

Cachexia — a wasting syndrome when a sufferer loses weight

Causalgia — severe burning pain in a limb caused by injury

Cerebral palsy — a movement disorder caused by brain damage in infancy

Cervical dystonia — is where the neck muscles contract involuntarily, causing awkward posture of the head and neck.

Chiari malformation — where the lower part of the brain pushes on the spinal cord causing a range of symptoms including headaches, double vision and nausea

Chronic inflammatory demyelinating polyneuropathy — a neurological disorder that causes nerve swelling or inflammation

Chronic renal failure needing dialysis — kidney failure

Chronic traumatic encephalopathy — a type of dementia associated with repeated blows to the head. Sometimes known as being 'punch-drunk'

Complex regional pain syndrome (CRPS) - a chronic pain condition that often affects one limb after injury

Decompensated cirrhosis — alcohol related liver disease

Ehlers-Danlos syndrome — a group of disorders that affect connective tissues causing loose joints

End-of-life care

Fibrous dysplasia — a condition present at birth that affects bone growth and development. Affected bones are weak and misshapen

Hepatitis C — a form of viral hepatitis transmitted in infected blood, causing chronic liver disease

Hydrocephalus with intractable headaches — fluid on the brain that causes constant headaches

Inclusion body myositis — an inflammatory muscle disease affecting older adults

Interstitial cystitis — a chronic bladder health issue, with the feeling of pain and pressure in the bladder area. Along with this pain are lower urinary tract symptoms which have lasted for more than six weeks, without having an infection or other clear causes

Intractable migraine — persistent, chronic, migraine that fails to respond to traditional treatment

Lupus — an autoimmune disease where your body's defence system attacks your own tissues. Symptoms include inflammation, swelling, and damage to the joints, skin, kidneys, blood, heart, and lungs

Mitochondrial disease — mitochondria act like batteries, powering cells, but in mitochondrial disease the DNA does not fuel cells fully, causing muscle wasting and weakness

Muscular dystrophy — an incurable muscle weakening disease

Nail-patella syndrome — a genetic disorder resulting in poorly developed nails and knee-caps

Post laminectomy syndrome with chronic radiculopathy — chronic pain following back surgery and a condition due to a compressed spinal nerve that causes pain, numbness, tingling or weakness. Most common in the lower back and neck.

Psoriasis — a skin disease marked by red itchy, scaly patches

Psoriatic arthropathy — a type of arthritis suffered by some people with psoriasis

Rheumatoid arthritis — a chronic autoimmune disease, causing painful inflammation in the joints

Sickle cell disease — a genetic blood disorder caused by faulty red blood cells

Sjogren's syndrome — an immune system disorder characterised by dry eyes and mouth

Spinal stenosis — is a narrowing of the spaces within the spine, which puts pressure on the spinal nerves

Spinocerebellar ataxia (SCA) — is a progressive, degenerative, genetic disease which affects co-ordination

Syringomyelia — a rare disorder where a cyst forms in your spinal cord

Tarlov cyst syndrome — fluid filled cysts found mostly at the base of the spine

Admittance into hospice care

Trigeminal neuralgia — severe facial pain

Then in **California**, it is allowed for:

- Any other chronic or persistent medical symptom that substantially limits the ability of the person to conduct one or more major life activities (as defined by the Americans with

Disabilities Act of 1990) or, if not alleviated, may cause serious harm to the patient's safety or physical or mental health

And in **Washington DC**, the Health Regulation and Licensing Administration say it can be used for:

- Any other condition that is chronic, cannot be effectively treated by ordinary medical measures, or,

- Any condition for which treatment with medical marijuana would be beneficial, as determined by the patient's physician

The bottom line is, medical cannabis can be really effective for many symptoms and conditions, and it is often worth trying, with a prescription, to see whether symptoms improve.

CHAPTER 4

How to take medical cannabis

With every condition, you need to start with a high CBD, full extract product. Full extract means that although it's high in CBD, it includes other cannabinoids like CBN, CBG and CBC for example. If you're not getting the desired effect then add in THC, little by little until you find the right balance. The United Patients Alliance, a British lobbying group, have a list of manufacturers they on their website[lviii]. And CBDoilreview.org in the US have a list on their website[lix].

Sensible precautions

- It makes sense to try medical cannabis at home first, rather than when you have to be at work or at a social engagement.

- As with all dosing, it is best to start low and work your way up, and/or start with a CBD rich concentrate before increasing the THC content. This helps to root out any side effects that might affect work or socialising.

- THC can impair driving performance so avoid driving or operating machinery if you feel drowsy or disorientated.

- Non-psychoactive cannabinoids like CBD do not carry a risk with driving.

- There are four main ways to take medical cannabis: smoking, vaping, eating, or orally as a capsule or oil or tincture taken under the tongue.

Smoking

- The recreational way to take cannabis is to smoke it, but adding it to tobacco and rolling a big joint to puff on for medical reasons makes no sense because of the links between tobacco and lung cancer

- In my view, the evidence is against cannabis smoke causing a higher risk of lung cancer when it is smoked without tobacco. In fact, some studies have shown that compounds found in the cannabis smoke actually have an anti-cancer effect

- Nevertheless, smoking cannot be recommended for medical purposes and the November 2018 British government regulations still outlaw smoking, whilst they allow any other form of taking the medicine. There are plenty of other, safer ways to get medical cannabis into your system

Vaporisation — Vaping

- Vaporisation basically involves a prescribed cannabis flower or cannabis concentrate being heated to a temperature that releases the cannabinoids, THC and terpenes, but not heated enough to release the undesirable parts of the flower, such as tar

- The temperature to release the cannabinoids and terpenes is between 180°C (360°F) to 210°C (410°F), but the temperature reached when smoking is far higher — 220°C (430°F) and more

- Vaporising is definitely healthier than smoking and acts to preserve the unique flavours and effects of the cannabis flower or concentrate, whereas smoking will burn off some of the naturally occurring components

- Vaporising is often preferred to smoking; people feel they get a better and more satisfying effect

There are two main types of vaporising equipment – conduction equipment and convection equipment:

Conductive vaporisers

In conductive vaporisers, the dried flower or the extract is placed directly onto an electrically heated surface or hot plate. Once the plate reaches the desired temperature, you inhale the vapour. The most common temperature to heat it to is around 190°C (375°F) to 210°C (410°F). The manufacturer will advise which is best.

Convection vaporisers

With convection, the cannabis doesn't actually come into contact with the heating element, the cannabinoid and terpene vapour are released by heating air. Hot air passes through the cannabis when you suck through a tube, delivering the cannabinoid and terpene vapour. Many vaporisers now allow the temperature to be adjusted.

The importance of temperature

Different cannabinoids and terpenes evaporate at different temperatures so the medical (and recreational) effect can be varied by varying the temperature. THC, for example, evaporates at 157°C (314.6°F) whereas the terpene myrcene evaporates at the higher temperature of about 168°C (334.4°F).

Adjusting the temperature can mean the vapour has slightly different components. You will notice different smells at different temperatures. Lower ones, release terpenes like the smell of pine forests — alpha-pinene — and the wood spice of caryophyllene — while at higher temperatures, the smells like coriander and orange from the terpene linalool are more noticeable.

Some people say that THC vaporised at low temperatures has a slightly less marked effect than the THC vaporised at higher temperatures. Some other minor cannabinoids also have higher vaporising temperatures.

Table top and pen vaporisers
There are many commercial vaporisers on the market which makes the whole process remarkably easy. They come as a pen, as a portable vape, which is slightly larger than a pen, and as a small desk top box that needs to be plugged in. In the end, it's a matter of personal preference.

Table top vaporisers
Table top vaporisers suit people whose medical needs are always going to be met at home. The best known, and most expensive vaporiser, which costs around £290, ($550) is the Volcano by Storz and Bickel, but you can pay as little as £20 ($25) for a table top vaporiser.

Vape pens
If you need medical cannabis outside the home, then a portable vape pen is better. Some vape pens use a screw in sealed cylindrical cartridge, such as Just CBD's Signature cartridge[ix] or Koi Naturals CBD Cartridge,[xi] both available in the US, while Dank Vapes[xii] sell in the UK. Many come with a standard 510 thread (that's 10 threads on the cylinder at 0.5 mm per thread. It's pretty standard but worth asking when you buy) so they fit into most vape pens.

Others have cylinders which can be filled directly with oil which you can either get on prescription or buy from shops where cannabis oil is sold legally. At the moment, in the UK, there is a very limited choice of sealed cartridges. If you need to vape, then getting a prescription for dried flower or full extract oil from a specialist is the more likely option.

Capsules and Oils

In medical terms, particularly in the new markets, many countries insist that medicinal cannabis products are sold only in the form of oils or capsules, and in most countries, capsule or oil formulations are most likely to be sold by leading, reputable producers.

Capsules

- A capsule is simply the oil wrapped up in an easy to swallow gelatine parcel. The advantage of the capsule route is that it makes the dose easy to control, as reputable manufacturers will state the number of milligrams of the cannabinoid, (usually THC and CBD) per ml, or drop, on the label

- Doctors find it easier to prescribe them too. If the prescription is 200mg a day for example, the doctor can prescribe one 50mg capsule to be taken four times a day. Understandably, doctors prefer to prescribe specific dosages rather than the less certain method of a weight of dried flower. It also feels more professional to the doctor and more like taking a medicine rather than a recreational drug

- Capsules are absorbed through the gastrointestinal system and are then metabolised by the liver, before being absorbed into the blood stream. The bioavailability of capsules is often less than oil drops and sometimes one needs a slightly higher dose of capsule medicine than oil medicine

Cannabis Oils

Many oils are taken by simply dropping the liquid under the tongue. This way, some of the oil is absorbed directly into the blood stream and starts to act quickly on a similar timescale to vaping or smoking. Your doctor should be able to advise.

Ratio of CBD to THC in capsules and oils

Manufacturers, who produce their products to Good Manufacturing Practice standards, have a variety of capsules or oils available with different ratios of CBD to THC. Usually, they produce a high CBD, low THC product, as well as a high THC, low CBD product and a range of more balanced THC to CBD ratios. A good manufacturer also notes the presence of other minor cannabinoids and displays the terpene profile so that the patient can pick the type and style that best suits them. The oils should come with a dropper.

Edibles
Activation of THC - decarb your cannabis before cooking with it

When you smoke or vape cannabis, the heat activates the THC naturally. This doesn't happen if you sprinkle it raw into food. If you cook with it, the heat from the cooking process will activate the THC as long as the cooking temperature reaches 120°C (250°F) or above. If you want to use it in oils or butter, or any food that doesn't need cooking. You need to decarb your cannabis.

- The technical term for this is decarboxylate, shortened to decarb. If your cannabis has not been decarbed, you will not feel the full effect of it

- If cannabis isn't properly decarbed before cooking, bacteria can grow in your tinctures, butters and oils. The decarboxylating process destroys bacteria

- Cannabis begins decarbing at about 120°C (250°F). The process takes about 30 to 45 minutes and can easily be done in an oven

- Some people decarb at lower temperatures for longer, which should preserve the terpenes better

- Medical oils and capsules will already be decarboxylated, so this really only applies to a prescription of dried flower

- Place your cannabis flower on a sheet of baking parchment placed on a baking tray

- Break any large pieces up and make sure it's in a thin layer. If it's too crowded, it won't dry out properly

- Check after 30 minutes. If it's light to medium brown in colour and dry, it's ready, if not, put it back in the oven for another 5 to 10 minutes. Remove, leave to cool and store in a sealed bag or jar

Cookies, breads and brownies

Edibles are becoming increasingly popular in countries where medical (and recreational) cannabis is legal and taking cannabis in food or drink is one of the favourite ways to take it. Any food product can be infused with cannabis extracts, but it is usually found in cookies, bread and chocolate brownies.

The American company SpeedWeed[lxiii] offers 49 edible cannabis products: cookies, chewy sweets and snack bars and they have gluten free and vegan-friendly varieties. In the UK, options to buy ready-made edibles are limited, but Hemp Elf[lxiv] sell chocolate and gummy sweets.

There are many cannabis cook books like *Herb,* by American chefs Melissa Parks and Laurie Wolf, and if you want a cannabis cocktail you'll find plenty of recipes in the book, *Cannabis Cocktails, Mocktails & Tonics* by mixologist Warren Bobrow.

Cannabis butters, oils, wines and beers

You can cook any food with a cannabis butter, or a cannabis infused oil and you can also drink cannabis wine and beer. There is cannabis sparkling water — produced by the Heineken company — and fruit juice infused with cannabis. A whole new culinary world opens up.

Cannabis is not water friendly —- it prefers to be dissolved in fatty oils. There are techniques, called nano emulsification, that effectively make cannabis mix with water. This avoids the 'salad dressing' effect, where oil and water don't mix. We will no doubt see many more cannabis infused drinks in the future.

Effects of edible cannabis

The effect of an edible is not as certain in terms of dosage and time frame to take effect, as vaping or taking a capsule or liquid. Vaping effects are almost immediate but eating or drinking takes one to two hours to kick in. It makes the dosage a little harder to control and there is a risk with a delayed effect; individuals who are not used to the process may feel that there has been no effect and take more food or drink. This puts you at risk of taking too much.

The bioavailability of the medical cannabis is also less with edibles, as food and drink have to pass from the stomach into the gut, where they are then absorbed and processed by the liver. The liver filters out some of the cannabis or converts it to breakdown products to be excreted, usually in the urine. The effect is less certain than absorbing the cannabis straight into the blood stream by vaping or placing the oil under the tongue.

The one advantage of edibles is that, although the effect is delayed, it lasts longer (several hours longer usually), which helps people suffering with conditions like chronic pain.

Cannabis Lotions, Balms, Oils and Topicals

- Topicals are cannabis infused lotions, balms or oils that are absorbed through the skin; very useful for localised pain relief or inflammation

- Other forms of topical administration are increasing, such as skin pain patches, which give a longer lasting effect

- Topical application does not generally induce euphoria, or at least a much less intense euphoric feeling that you would get from smoking or ingesting cannabis. This is because the absorption is just to the local area and not, or at least very little, is absorbed into the blood stream and into the brain

Other Forms of Medical Cannabis

Rectal suppositories can be particularly helpful for those with a painful mouth or throat. Vaginal pessaries can be used for localised gynaecological conditions, or as an alternative way of absorption. They are also meant to enhance the sexual experience! According to an informal poll by the magazine *Psychology Today*,[lxv] 67 per cent of respondents felt that cannabis enhanced their sex lives.

CHAPTER 5

Side effects

The information in this chapter about side effects comes from many good quality studies and medical cannabis trials.

SPECIAL NOTE: Children using medical cannabis for epilepsy

- Some parents worry about the effect of THC on the developing brain in children, but the evidence of harm is thin and controversial

- It's always worth considering the risk/benefit ratio. What is more likely to harm: steroids, opioids, other strong drugs, or medical cannabis?

- Side effects from epilepsy drugs can be harsh and damaging. According to the NHS, common side effects caused by anti-epileptic drugs (AEDs) include drowsiness, lack of energy, agitation, headache, tremor, hair loss or unwanted hair growth, swollen gums and rashes

- Most of the studies have looked at adolescents using regular street cannabis and there is some evidence that those adolescents suffer some long-term cognitive problems

- Other studies, where the control group has used alcohol, show no bad effects

- In my view, the risk of THC in young children, in small doses and counterbalanced by large doses of CBD, is minimal

SPECIAL NOTE: Pregnancy and breastfeeding

- Cannabis is best avoided in pregnancy

- There have been no proper studies into the effect on the growing foetus, but some case studies suggest a link with various problems, such as smaller birth weight and preterm delivery

- In 2018, a study by the University of Colorado, Denver, US[lxvi] recently concluded that more work was needed to know definitely, but advised against using cannabis while pregnant or while breastfeeding

Medical trials

In medical cannabis trials, side effects are often measured in terms of the drop-out rate from the studies. Cannabis studies enjoy a low drop-out rate, mostly less than 10 per cent. Compare that to drop-out rates of around 33 per cent in opioid trials.

Likelihood of side effects or adverse events — the odds ratio

A paper[lxvii] published in 2015 by European and American researchers, looked at adverse events across 62 cannabis studies. The authors listed the top 20 individual adverse events with what is called an odds ratio (OR) — a measure of the increase or decrease in the chance of side effects compared to a placebo drug.

These are the leading side effects across the studies. Remember most of these problems occur with high THC medicines and CBD medicines have fewer side effects.:

TOP 20 ADVERSE EVENTS - ODDS RATIO (OR)

- Disorientation – OR 5.41 – or a 5.41 increased chance of disorientation compared to placebo
- Dizziness – 5.09
- Euphoria – 4.08
- Confusion – 4.03
- Drowsiness – 3.68
- Dry mouth – 3.5
- Sleepiness – 2.83
- Balance problems – 2.62
- Hallucinations – 2.19
- Nausea – 2.08
- Paranoia – 2.05
- Lack of energy – 2.03
- Lethargy – 2.03
- Fatigue – 2
- Anxiety – 1.98
- Vomitting – 1.67
- Diarrhoea – 1.65
- Depression – 1.32
- Psychosis – 1.09

Comparison with other drugs

- The OR for suffering respiratory problems from opioids is OR 4.0, according to a study published in the journal _Anaesthesiology_ in 2018,[lxviii] which gives some perspective

- The list of short-term effects might look daunting but compare them to medicines that come with a 'black box' warning. A black box warning means that side effects caused by these drugs can be fatal

- Drugs prescribed for chronic pain like morphine or fentanyl, which can cause severe constipation, itchy skin, nausea, vomiting, problems breathing, dizziness, dry mouth and drowsiness, can also cause death with overdose

- As can insomnia and anxiety drugs from the benzodiazepine (benzo) group like Xanax and Valium.

- No medical cannabis has a black box warning

- For most people taking medicinal cannabis, the effects are either non-existent, or mild and not a problem

How long do side effects last?

- Every drug has side effects and cannabis is no exception

- They can be split into two camps — short-term side effects: that last while the drug is active in the body, and long-term side effects, as a result of prolonged use

- How you take cannabis will influence the side effects that you experience

- Effects are stronger, but last less time, from vaporising or taking drops under the tongue, whereas they are usually milder and longer lasting, from taking capsules or edibles. Effects very much depend on the dose.

Short term effects

The higher the THC content the more side effects are involved, although relaxing CBD counteracts some of the euphoric effects of THC. CBD dominant strains have less side effects than THC dominant strains.

In fact, CBD is remarkably safe, although a small number of people, about 3 per cent, are very sensitive to cannabis and may get side effects at normal doses but not at smaller doses. Others can tolerate very high doses of cannabis with very few side effects. People vary in their reactions, like they would with any drug.

Long Term Effects

Those opposing the legalisation of cannabis, even for medical purposes, say there are long-term problems with cannabis use. Most studies into the long-term problems have been carried out with recreational users taking unknown quality and quantities of cannabis, usually THC dominant, over a long period of time. This is a different population from medical users, although it is worth looking at some of the problems noted after long term recreational cannabis use. These are:

Psychosis

In the UK, the NHS website[lxix] warns that medical cannabis can cause psychosis. They say: 'There is evidence that regular cannabis use increases your risk of developing a psychotic illness such as schizophrenia.' This information is based on studies with recreational users rather than those taking medical cannabis, but because there is a small risk, we've included details here.

- The risk of cannabis causing schizophrenia or psychosis is very low, but is an issue for some people, particularly those with a family history of schizophrenia

- Anyone who has had, or is suffering, a schizophrenic illness or psychosis should avoid medical cannabis

- This is particularly true in young people and especially young men

- The problem is caused by THC, whereas CBD may work as an anti-psychotic

It's worth looking at the science. A study in the journal *Human Molecular Genetics*[lxx] published in 2017, found that THC increased the risk of psychiatric disorders like schizophrenia in adolescent recreational users although the issue of cannabis use, and the onset of schizophrenia and/or psychotic symptoms is complex. Many other factors should be considered, such as social class, other drug use and 'reverse causality': where an individual starts to use cannabis as a means of coping with low mood or mental health issues. Cannabis use cannot be attributed as the cause when the illness may have been there before.

Some say that the association with psychosis is over-estimated and a 2009 paper[lxxi] from researchers at the University of Bristol, UK, showed how many recreational cannabis users would need to stop the habit in order to prevent one case of schizophrenia or psychosis. For men, aged 20 to 24, they found 2,800 heavy cannabis users would need to stop the habit to prevent one case of schizophrenia, while 10,000 light users would need to stop. For women, aged 20 to 24, 7,700 heavy users would need to stop and a remarkable 29,000 for light users.

Effects on the heart

- A reasonably common complication of high THC cannabis, is a rapid heart rate, which whilst uncomfortable, is usually not an issue

- Obviously, in some people with cardiac disease, a sudden increase in heart rate can be a problem

- Some studies have shown an increase in heart attack after cannabis use, but others have not and some even show a lower death rate after heart attack in marijuana users

- A review by Indian and American researchers, found that heart attack or stroke is a very rare complication

Dependence

- In 2007, *The Lancet*,[lxxii] a well-known British medical journal, published a scale to assess the harm of some drugs, both medical and recreational

- Heroin topped the list, followed by cocaine, tobacco, barbiturates (sedatives), alcohol, benzodiazepines (sleeping and anti-anxiety pills) and amphetamines (stimulants)

- Cannabis was eighth on the list with a dependence rate of 9 per cent, compared with a 15 per cent rate for alcohol, 17 per cent for cocaine, 23 per cent for heroin and a huge 32 per cent for tobacco

Dependence is formally defined by the American Psychiatric Association (APA) in their *Diagnostic and Statistical Manual of Mental Disorders* (DSM)[lxxiii] as: "A cluster of physiological, behavioural, and cognitive phenomena in which the use of a substance, or class of substances, takes on a much higher priority for a given individual than other behaviours that once had greater value." That's a long-winded way of saying that dependence is a constant strong desire, or compulsion, to take cannabis or any other drug.

The risk is relatively small but can be an issue for some people. For medical use, with a good quality product and a low THC ratio, the risk of dependency is likely to be smaller than the risk to recreational users. Dependence is more of a problem in adolescence and early adulthood; the younger the age starting cannabis, the higher the risk of dependency. If dependency does become a problem, then seek specialist advice from an addiction service.

Excessive use

- Excessive use of cannabis can cause some cognitive difficulties, such as short-term problems with attention, concentration, memory and decision making

- Acute intoxication is unusual, and if it occurs, is usually mild and short-lived

- In long term medical use, researchers at The Scripps Research Institute, in California, US, said in 2011,[lxxiv] that cognitive problems last several hours, or even several days, after use has ended, but a 2018 study with over 2,000 adolescents and young adults, by the University of Pennsylvania in Philadelphia, US,[lxxv] shows no problems in the medium or long term

- A good quality review of papers in 2018, also by researchers at the University of Pennsylvania, Philadelphia, US, looked at 69 studies covering over 2000 cannabis users (average age 20 years) and found a small short-term negative effect on cognition, but after 72 hours abstinence there was no longer any effect

- A long-term study of Sativex in 2012,[lxxvi] showed no long-term cognitive problems after at least one year of usage, although 14 per cent stopped because of side effects

What happens if you take too much cannabis?

- There is no evidence that anyone has died from a cannabis overdose. It is a remarkably safe drug
- If you take too much, particularly of the THC products, there is no need to panic as the effects of the excess high will wear off over time
- Most overdoses occur after eating edibles because of the delay in effect of up to a couple of hours. People get over-enthusiastic looking for results and can take too much
- With THC, it's unlikely you will notice any side effects until you take a product with a level of 8 per cent to 10 per cent THC
- There is no guarantee that you will suffer but if you do, the side effects from THC can last between four and six hours
- Severity of the side effects depends on how much has been taken and can include increased heart rate, anxiety and panic attacks
- In the short term, you might experience difficulties like hallucinations and delusions, a loss of personal identity, poor coordination, difficulty speaking, shortness of breath, shaking and sweating, sudden high blood pressure with headache, or you might suffer from paranoia

Sometimes, in a cannabis overdose situation, other substances are implicated as well, such as other drugs or alcohol. These may need specific treatment, but, if there is just cannabis involved, there is no need to worry unless the reaction is particularly bad; then go to hospital.

Doctors may treat various symptoms with calming drugs for anxiety, or drugs to reduce pulse rate.

Time is the best healer, as well as drinking lots of water and staying hydrated. Eating something can help too. CBD is known to counteract the effect of THC, so you can try CBD as a rescue remedy or antidote. The basic message is to wait and sleep it off.

Cannabis allergy

- Genuine allergy to cannabis is so unusual that there are no figures recording numbers who have suffered, but it can occur. It is more likely that the allergy is to the oil used in the delivery system; for example, an oil like almond or coconut

- Itchy eyes, asthma, facial swelling or rashes have been described but mainly in those who smoke or vape cannabis

- Occasionally, passive cannabis smokers can suffer respiratory problems, like with passive tobacco smoke

- It is rare but people with allergies to peach, banana, apple, nuts or tomatoes can also be allergic to cannabis. This is called the cannabis-fruit/vegetable syndrome. The best way to stop this is to avoid cannabis

Cannabis hyperemesis syndrome is a rare complication, mainly occurring in people using a high THC street product. Symptoms are severe nausea, vomiting and stomach cramp. Rehydration may be needed in hospital. It can be helped, oddly, by a hot shower.

CHAPTER 6

Drug interactions

How your body processes medical cannabis

It's useful to understand how your body deals with medical cannabis as it helps to understand how other prescription drugs might affect how it works.

All drugs have to reach your liver at some point. The liver is your body's toxin filter whose job it is to get rid of as many nasty substances from your blood as possible. It's the sole responsibility of enzymes in your liver, called cytochromes, to clean your internal house and get rid of toxic substances.

Drugs, once they have done what they are supposed to do, cannot be allowed to build up in your body. The liver will not allow them to be swept under the carpet, and enzymes in the liver try their best to remove them. Drugs are not part of the body's permanent decor and have to go. To do this, one of your 60 cytochromes goes into action every time it comes across any kind of drug — herbal or chemical — breaking it down and usually sending it to the kidneys to excrete.

Individual sensitivity

- Our bodies react very differently and some of us have more efficient livers than others. This makes a difference to how much medical cannabis — and other drugs — we can tolerate
- It also influences how strong, or weak, the effect of those substances is

- The reason some people are more sensitive to THC is that the cytochrome responsible for breaking down THC is less efficient in them. More THC reaches the blood stream and major organs, having a stronger effect

- The specific cytochromes responsible for breaking down THC have great *Star Wars* style names: CYP2C9 and CYP3A4

- In some people, these enzymes don't work too efficiently and so those people need smaller doses of THC

Prescription drug interactions

- A common question is: "Can I take cannabis when I am taking other medicines?" The basic answer is yes, in most circumstances

- Cannabis has a few interactions with prescription medicine, but, most of the time, they are not a major problem and you can continue taking your pills

- In some cases, you can actually reduce some, like opioids and anticonvulsant drugs as we've discussed, and it may be possible to reduce anti-anxiety drugs

- It is worth explaining the mechanics of what can happen, so that if something doesn't feel quite right, you and your doctor can work out what is going on.

- See below:

Some prescription drugs cause the body to get rid of THC slower so you may feel the effects for longer. There is little evidence that taking these drugs at the same time as medical cannabis containing THC, leads to any significant problem.

- They include amiodarone (used to treat heart rhythm problems)

- The antacid cimetidine

- The antibiotics cotrimoxazole and metronidazole

- The antidepressants fluoxetine and fluvoxamine (fluvoxamine is also used to treat OCD and anxiety disorders)

- The anti-fungal drug fluconazole

- Ketoconazole, another anti-fungal drug, inhibits the enzyme CYP3A4, which would increase the concentration of THC in your body

- Other drugs that hamper CYP3A4 include the antibiotics clarithromycin and erythromycin

- Cyclosporine, an immunosuppressant drug often used in rheumatoid arthritis, psoriasis or Crohn's disease

- Verapamil, taken for high blood pressure, angina or other heart rhythm disorders

- The antibiotic rifampicin *speeds up* the action of CYP3A4, so, THC levels are reduced by around 20 per cent to 40 per cent. This means less effect from the THC

This is not a definitive list, but these are the main drugs that can theoretically affect THC levels in your blood stream. Your prescribing doctor should know if any medication you are taking could cause problems.

Effects of cannabis on other drugs

Levels of warfarin (a blood thinning agent) can be increased in people taking cannabis. If you are taking warfarin, then be more careful about monitoring the amount you are taking.

Sometimes cannabis can cause an enzyme called CYP1A2 to breakdown drugs faster. Some drugs known to be affected are:

• Theophylline, used in lung disease and asthma

• The anti-psychotic drug chlorpromazine

• People taking the anti-epileptic drug clobazam should be vigilant as clobazam levels can increase when taking medical cannabis, particularly CBD This can cause drowsiness. If this happens, then it is worth having a blood test to check the level of clobazam and taking a smaller dose if needed

Cytochromes and CBD

There are a couple of cytochromes that affect CBD — CYP3A4, and one we haven't mentioned before called CYP2C19. People taking the anti-fungal drug ketoconazole show increased concentrations in the blood of CBD by about two-fold; as the enzymes are slowed down, CBD increases, as it is not broken down as quickly.

It has the opposite effect on the antibiotic rifampicin, and CBD levels are reduced by about 50 per cent as the enzymes are stimulated. This is slightly less important in terms of side effects, as CBD doesn't have psychoactive properties, but a change in plasma levels can affect its medicinal properties.

Pharmacodynamic interactions -- how one drug affects another and the side effects

There are other interactions, called pharmacodynamic interactions. This means, for example, that if you are taking a drug that causes high heart rate, taking medical cannabis containing THC, which can also cause a high heart rate, can mean that the high heart rate increases more than usual.

The best known pharmacodynamic issue is the nervous system depressant effect (drowsiness and sleepiness) of alcohol, which mixed with some indica varieties of cannabis, cause additional drowsiness or sleepiness.

If you have any doubts at all then consult your doctor. You should definitely tell your doctor if you take medical (or recreational) cannabis while on any prescription medicine.

CHAPTER 7

Legal situation around the globe

By February 2019, 47 countries had some form of legalised medical cannabis available on prescription. That figure is increasing rapidly.

Each country approaches the issue of medical cannabis differently and most have had to bring in new legislation as existing medical drug approval does not readily apply to the cannabis plant. It is just too complicated, with so many cannabinoids and terpenes, most of which, if not all, may have some medicinal value.

In June 2018, Professor Dame Sally Davies, Chief Medical Officer and Chief Medical Advisor to the UK Government, produced a review[lxxvii] of cannabis. She recommended that cannabis-based medicinal products should be moved out of a Schedule 1 classification (of the Misuse of Drugs Regulations 2001), as Schedule 1 drugs have little or no therapeutic value. Taking cannabis out of Schedule 1 makes medical cannabis more readily prescribable by doctors. This happened in the UK on 1 November 2018.

In the US, the first state legalise medical cannabis was California, in 1966. Now in the majority of states doctors can prescribe it or recommend it.

Which countries legally allow medical cannabis?

- Some countries allow only CBD, usually with only very low amounts of THC (usually less than 0.2 per cent) which comes from industrial hemp. That varies though. Switzerland, for example, allows up to 1 per cent of THC in their CBD products.

- Other countries allow CBD but do not allow it to be sold as a medicine only as a food supplement.
- Some countries allow THC products but may put an upper limit on THC content. Mexico has a 1 per cent THC limit.
- Some countries restrict the conditions in which it can be prescribed or restrict those who can prescribe it. In some countries, it can only be recommended and not prescribed by doctors.
- Many countries have decriminalised cannabis so possession for medical or recreational use is not a criminal offence but a minor offence, so still not legal.
- Other places simply have not changed the law but tolerate cannabis use. This can happen in different parts of the same country. Catalonia in Spain, for example, is more tolerant than the rest of Spain, cannabis being allowed in private member clubs in Barcelona.
- In Holland, the well-known cannabis cafés allow recreational use, but it is still illegal other than for medicinal use.
- In the US, the government says each state can decide on its own law. Although they have not made it federally legal, states are not prevented from deciding whether it should be available on prescription, without a prescription, with limited THC or totally banned. Cannabis cannot be transported across state lines.

Pharmaceutical cannabis products

Pharmaceutical cannabis products which are licensed drugs and mostly legal:

- nabiximols (Sativex)
- nabilone (Cesamet)

- dronabinol (Marinol and Syndros)
- cannabidiol (Epidiolex)

In the USA:

- Epidiolex is now legal and approved by the US Food and Drug Administration agency (FDA)
- Synthetic nabilone and dronabinol are also legally approved but not Sativex!

In the UK:

- Sativex is allowed but only doctors in Wales can prescribe it because of cost. It is available on private prescription.
- Epidiolex and dronabinol are not yet licensed but nabilone is.

In other words, there's no global consensus in the US, or around the world.

World Health Organisation (WHO) and other regulatory bodies

- The WHO says that CBD may have medicinal properties and has: "...no public health related problems."
- The World Anti-Doping Agency (WADA) has removed CBD from its banned substance list.
- The United Nations (UN) is now looking at whether the Single Convention Scheduling, is appropriate for medical cannabis. (The Single Convention on Narcotic Drugs was a treaty put together in 1961 to prohibit the production and supply of specific drugs. It has four schedules of controlled substances which are decided by the WHO and The Commission on Narcotic Drugs. Cannabis is currently

listed in schedules I and IV alongside opium, morphine and cocaine, while hemp is excluded.)

Travelling with cannabis

Check the legal situation at your destination and even the situation when transiting through an international airport. Dubai, for example, has very strict drug laws. Even transiting through the airport may cause problems with cannabis medicine legally obtained in one country and travelling to another legal jurisdiction. You can get around this by buying it at the final destination or sending it ahead, as long as it is legal in that destination.

How to find out the situation in any given country?

For global information on THC, start with the Wikipedia website called Legality of Cannabis[lxxviii] and be sure to cross check the information with the appropriate country before travelling.

For global information on CBD, check the website Supplements in Review[lxxix]. Cross check again. Remember, you need to check the situation by state in the US.

COUNTRIES ALLOWING MEDICAL CANNABIS WITH THC AND CBD*

EUROPE	Austria Belgium Croatia Cyprus Czech Republic, Denmark Estonia Finland France (restricted), Georgia Germany	Greece Ireland Israel Italy Luxembourg Macedonia Malta Netherlands Norway Poland Portugal Romania San Marino	Slovenia Spain Switzerland Turkey United Kingdom (can only be prescribed by specialists)
SOUTH AMERICA	Argentina Chile	Columbia Peru	Uruguay
AUSTRALASIA AND OCEANA	Australia	New Zealand	Vanuatu
ASIA	North Korea (possibly yes, but please check)	South Korea	Sri Lanka (very limited)
AFRICA	South Africa	Zimbabwe	

NORTH AMERICAN COUNTRIES WHERE MEDICAL

CANNABIS IS LEGAL

AND NORTH AMERICA BY STATE

NORTH AMERICA	Canada Grenadines	Jamaica Mexico	Saint Vincent
NORTH AMERICA BY STATE			
Totally prohibited	Idaho Nebraska South Dakota	American Samoa	US Virgin Islands
Available without prescription	Alaska California Colorado Maine Massachusetts	Michigan Nevada Oregon Vermont Washington	Washington DC, Northern Mariana Islands
Available with prescription	Arizona Arkansas Connecticut Delaware Florida Hawaii Illinois Louisiana Maryland	Minnesota Missouri Montana New Hampshire New Jersey New Mexico New York North Dakota	Ohio Oklahoma Pennsylvania Rhode Island Utah Virginia West Virginia Guam Puerto Rico
Available with limited THC content	Alabama Georgia Indiana Iowa Kansas	Kentucky Mississippi North Carolina South Carolina	Tennessee Texas Wyoming

*Worldwide situation

At the time of publishing, both tables give the most up-to-date list of countries allowing medical cannabis containing CBD and THC in some form. Please check for updates.

CHAPTER 8

What to do if you want to take medical cannabis

So, you have got this far and hopefully, now understand a bit about cannabis and the endocannabinoid system, whether medicinal cannabis will suit you and if so what its effects, good and bad, might be. (If you want more detail, go to Part 2.)

You may decide it's not for you. Fair enough. Or, you may decide you would like to try it. If so, what are the next steps?

Is what you want to buy legal where you live?

- Find out if it's legal and available. Is it legal in your country? (see page 85 and 86). Cannabis including strains with THC, is legal in 47 countries around the world for medical use, but it is not legal everywhere. Other countries have legal CBD, but products containing THC, or perhaps more than a trace amount, are illegal. It is important to find out the legal position in your own country.

- Differentiate between CBD and THC containing products. Also remember that Sativex (nabiximols), nabilone (Cesamet), dronabinol (Marinol and Syndros) and cannabidiol (Epidiolex) might be available even when natural plant full extract cannabis is not.

- CBD may be marketed as food supplement and not as a medicine.

Who will pay for it?

- Find out who pays for it. Assuming either CBD, and/or THC cannabis is legal, what then? The next stage is to find out whether it can be prescribed by a doctor, and whether it is available through that country's insurance systems or state medical systems.

- Are you eligible to receive a free prescription or will you need to pay for the medicine privately? The situation varies enormously.

Who can or will prescribe it?

- In the UK, from 1 November 2018, specialist doctors (hospital consultants) can legally prescribe cannabis derived medicinal products for any condition that in their opinion, can be treated with medical cannabis.

- Guidance has also been produced for doctors. Some doctors worry that if they prescribe against recommendations they will get into trouble with the General Medical Council (GMC), the public body in the UK responsible for regulating registered doctors. But if the doctor has taken a careful and thoughtful decision, based on a review of the evidence, they will not get into trouble. Refer to GMC and Department of Health guidance on these points (see Further reading).

- A hospital doctor will prescribe on a 'specials' system for unlicensed products, which may mean a bit of a delay in getting the medicine.

- In the UK, Sativex is prescribable by any doctor, but not readily available (except in Wales), because NICE has decided that it is not cost effective. It should be available on private prescription.

- Epidiolex is not yet available in the UK on normal prescription by a GP, although it is by a hospital doctor, but has now been licensed in the USA for some childhood drug-resistant epilepsies (Dravet syndrome and Lennox-Gastaut syndrome).

- Nabilone is prescribable in the UK, but for limited indications — nausea and vomiting during cancer chemotherapy — if other agents haven't worked.

- Dronabinol is not available in the UK.

- In the US the only prescription cannabis not available is Sativex. Epidiolex, Cesamet, Marinol and Syndros are all available.

- Find out who prescribes it. If it is legal and a doctor can prescribe, or at least recommend it, then the next port of call is your local doctor or physician. Most doctors in the UK have limited knowledge when it comes to medical cannabis. They may be supportive but are unwilling to make recommendations, simply because they do not understand the plant and know how, or what, to recommend. They are better informed in the US and Canada.

- The UK has formed a Medical Cannabis Clinicians Society (MCCS) and launched a teaching programme for doctors (although available to anyone free online). You can look at The Academy of Medical Cannabis for training modules.

- In Germany, only 2 per cent of doctors are prepared to prescribe. Hopefully, this situation will not last for many more years as cannabis becomes more widely available, and medical cannabis societies and medical education programmes become more widespread. The medical profession will eventually catch up.

- The US will vary by state. Check the situation in your state.

Be your own doctor

- Be your own doctor. Your own research may well be the most reliable source of information. Do not be afraid to challenge your doctor and present your research. This book, and more academic articles and books listed at the end of this chapter, may help.

- In countries where dispensaries are available to the public, chatting to the 'bud tender' may offer an informed opinion, as in Canada. This is rather like asking your local pharmacist's advice on medicines, prior to a prescription by a doctor.

How to choose the right product for you

- How to choose the product? There is not one product that suits every person with one particular condition. It has to be a matter of trial and error. This is partly a reflection on the lack of scientific studies, but mainly a reflection on the enormous variability of the plant's contents and the balance between the different cannabinoids and terpenes. It is unlikely that we will ever have one particular strain that suits everyone with one specific condition. This book, or your doctor, or your bud tender, may have pointed you in a particular direction but can do no more than that.

- Obviously, the choice available to you depends on what products are available in your country. Hopefully, the licensed producers in your country will be controlled, in the sense of having quality products that are manufactured to specific quality standards with proper clear labelling. Try to use a product that is made to Good Manufacturing Practice standards, as this will guarantee quality and consistency. Check on the producer's website. Make sure labelling is clear and do not buy anything for medical use does not clarify what it contains.

- What to choose? As a general guide it is worth starting with a product that is relatively high in CBD, particularly if you are not used to taking cannabis. This approach will mean that you do not suffer any psychoactive effects. Most medicinal users are not seeking a psychoactive high but are looking for medicinal benefit.

- There are actually few medical conditions that respond to only high THC, and I would suggest those products are best avoided until higher CBD, or balanced products, have been tried. If we take pain, we know that both CBD and THC have painkilling effects. So, at first try a product with a relatively high CBD. If that doesn't help, move on to a product that has more balanced THC:CBD ratio, and if that doesn't help, then finally move to a product which is relatively high in THC.

How should you take your cannabis?

- What about the method of ingestion? This is a matter of choice and it will depend on what is allowed in your own country. Some countries only allow cannabis oils and

97

vaping or edibles for medicinal use are not legal. In the UK, smoking is not allowed, but other types of ingestion are acceptable legally on prescription. In the US, it varies from state to state so best to check.

- If you have a wide choice of ways to take medical cannabis, you can experiment with the method that best suits you. Some prefer under the tongue drops for a stronger effect, or an edible for longer term background relief. Some use more than one method to suit different circumstances, such as a quicker effect with vaping, on a background of a longer effect from capsules or edibles.

What should you take?

- What about dose? Doctors like prescribing a particular drug in a particular dose. However, this is difficult for cannabis. It is best to only use products that have clear labelling with the milligrams of a particular component clearly printed on the label. For example, 30mg CBD per ml, or 2mg THC per ml. If you note down what you take in milligrams, and also then note down the effect, this will enable a slightly more scientific approach to future dosing. All dosing should start low and only increase slowly at weekly intervals.

- In terms of CBD, a dose of around 20mg to 30mg may be reasonable to start, but can be slowly but steadily built up to, say, 100mg to 200mg, or even higher. Some children with epilepsy need up to 1000mg CBD, or more. This is only with pure CBD (Epidiolex). Pure products need much higher doses, usually at least five times as high as the full extract cannabis products which contain a variety of

98

cannabinoids and terpenes. Remember, that some people need only a small dose to be effective.

- THC is used in much lower milligram dosages and some people start at just 1mg per day, which can be slowly built up to say around 20mg to 30mg daily. As THC has more side effects and is more psychoactive, it would be very unwise to start with a high THC compound, particularly if you are new to cannabis.

- If you use a balanced strain of CBD to THC, make sure that the labelling is clear, such as a THC:CBD strain that tells you that there are 2mg per ml of THC and 100mg per ml of CBD in that particular strain. In some strains, there is a fixed ratio which may suit some people, but others prefer separate titration with a high CBD strain on the one hand, and a high THC strain on the other hand.

- Many labels simply carry a percentage, such as: 'cannabis oil with 20 per cent THC'. This is not very helpful labelling, because while 20 per cent THC oil is 'stronger' than a 10 per cent THC oil, this doesn't help you to determine how many milligrams of THC there are per ml and makes recording the dose and effect more difficult.

- Remember that no one has died of a cannabis overdose, and if you try the strains slowly and carefully, then it is unlikely to cause harm. Preferably, this should all be done in consultation with your doctor.

Drug interactions

- Drug Interactions. If you are already on some medication from your doctor, then it is important to discuss whether there is likely to be any interaction with those drugs if you start medical cannabis. Have a look through chapters 5 and 6 for this point.

- There are many more drugs than listed in that chapter, but once your doctor understands how cannabis interacts with the drug breakdown enzymes, they should be able to tell you whether the medication you are taking is likely to mix with cannabis, or whether you should not take cannabis, or whether you may need a dose adjustment of existing drugs, such as a reduction of clobazam in childhood epilepsy. If your doctor doesn't know, then they should be able to find out.

Side effects

- What about side effects? Cannabis is generally very safe but obviously there are side effects (see chapter 5), and as a general principle, if you find the side effects, particularly with the THC products, intolerable at a particular dose, then pull back one dose level. If, for example, you find unacceptable psychoactive effects at 25mg of THC, then drop back to 20mg THC and see if that reduces the side effects. It is all common sense and it is good to feel empowered that you are able to control your condition on your terms.

So, the messages are:

1. You need to be as knowledgeable as possible about medical cannabis and the endocannabinoid system, as it is likely that your doctor will have limited knowledge.

2. Work together with your doctor to discuss the best product, the best form of taking it, and the best dose. It is always trial and error with the cannabis plant, but the mantra is 'start low and go slow'.

3. Preferably, start with a high CBD strain as this will counteract any psychoactive effects of the THC.

4. Once you have found a mode of ingestion, and a dosage, and cannabis strain that suits you then if your country allows it, experiment around that dose level. Refine your needs with slightly different balances of the minor cannabinoids and terpenes.

Cannabis medicine is a very personal medicine but don't be afraid to try it out as many people find it hugely beneficial. Over to you.

PART 2

CHAPTER 9

History of cannabis

Cannabis, hashish, reefer, ganja, pot, weed, dope, marijuana, whacky baccy… rarely has a plant been given so many nicknames, around 1,200 in all. Its impact on society truly has been mind-bending because it has been put to so many uses, both therapeutic and recreational.

Cannabis has been around for longer than humans. We don't know exactly when the plant evolved but DNA studies suggest around 20 to 25 million years ago. The first definite trace is from fossilised cannabis pollen found in Siberia, dated over three quarters of a million years ago.

Early man almost certainly knew the plant and therefore probably knew its properties. He would have needed very little expertise to cultivate it. And although the fossil is from Siberia, it probably originated in Central Asia, where cannabis grows very easily.

At least as early as 4,000 BC, cannabis is recorded as ridding a body of parasites, removing blood clots and for its use as an anaesthetic.

In India alone, there are more than 50 words for cannabis, including ganja and bhang. The holy Hindu book, Atharvaveda, written around 900 BC, uses the word 'bhanga' that most believe to be cannabis. 'Bhang' is still used across South Asia as an edible preparation of cannabis, especially in the yoghurt drink bhang lassi. Meanwhile, the Buddha supposedly lived on one hemp seed per day during his ascetic period. Unlikely, but a good story that illustrated how highly thought of hemp was. Today, practitioners of Indian Ayurvedic medicine still use cannabis for pain, insomnia and loss of appetite.

According to Reginald Campbell Thompson, author of *The Assyrian Herbal*, one of the earliest nomadic tribes, the Scythians, who originated in Iran but migrated to Siberia and Central Asia, used cannabis infused steam for ritual purposes. They invaded Mesopotamia around 700 BC, and thereafter, a new word, translated as 'hemp', entered early literature.

A well-documented reference from 200 AD to 250 AD, is from ancient China in a book of classic herbal medicine called *Shén Nóng Běncāo Jing*, (available in translation by medical historian Dr Sabine Wilms, as *The Divine Farmer's Classic Materia Medica*) which says that it was used both as a food and for its psychoactive properties.

Spreading westwards

The use of cannabis spread slowly westwards. The Egyptian word for cannabis is shemshemet, and it appears in Ebers Papyrus, an Egyptian medical papyrus dated around 1550 BC. Egyptologist, Lise Manniche, noted in her book: *An Ancient Egyptian Herbal*, that cannabis was used for tumours and for complications in childbirth. Its use is also well described for headaches, particularly migraines, and as a muscle relaxant.

In ancient Greece and Rome, cannabis was used as a surgical anaesthetic and analgesic, for epilepsy, eye conditions and as an anti-anxiety drug. It was also used in wine for recreational purposes.

Further north, in a 9th century English herbarium cannabis is recommended as a treatment for wounds and "pain of the innards".

Europe — middle ages to modern

In Christian Europe, the priestly classes remained suspicious as cannabis offered a way to contact the 'spiritual world', a domain exclusive to them. In 1484, Pope Innocent VIII, labelled cannabis as an unholy sacrament and for centuries, it largely fell out of therapeutic use.

It was resurrected in 1839 by an Irish physician. William O'Shaughnessy published the first modern treatise in a reputable journal: *Transactions of the Medical and Physical Society of Bengal,* "...on the preparations of the Indian hemp or ganja (cannabis indica)". O'Shaunessy worked for the British East India company in the 1830s and observed Indian doctors using cannabis to treat their patients for a variety of conditions, including rheumatism, cholera, tetanus and epilepsy. His description of treating a baby girl with infantile convulsions, is ahead of its time, "...the child is now in enjoyment of robust health and has regained her natural plump and happy appearance."

In 1841, O'Shaughnessy returned to Britain bringing cannabis seeds with him enabling chemists to produce tinctures for general use by doctors, who found it highly effective and embraced it as a remedy. It is thought O'Shaughnessy suggested cannabis for Queen Victoria's menstrual pains. No one knows whether she tried it but if she did, she would have enjoyed considerable relief.

Although the use of cannabis was generally accepted in medical circles in British India, the East India Company became worried by its use amongst workers. To investigate, he Indian Hemp Drugs Commission was established and was instructed by the British Government to look into: "...the deleterious effects alleged to be produced by the abuse of ganja." But, despite a lengthy 3,000-page report published by the

Anglo-Indian committee in 1894, with testimonies from 1,200 doctors, army officers, clergy and other interested parties, it was concluded that with moderate use: "… the evil effects of ganja had been exaggerated."

Meanwhile, across the Atlantic, cannabis had established itself as a fashionable drug and towards the end of the century, oriental-style hashish parlours were popping up all over the United States.

In the late 19th and early 20th centuries, medical prescription of cannabis began to decline, replaced by new synthetic medicines such as aspirin and barbiturates: synthetic and single molecule medicines took over from what were now considered to be multi-molecule, crude plants.

The Start of International Control

In the early 20th century, many governments became concerned about the international opium trade. Attempts to control the trade were made at conventions in Shanghai in 1909, and the Hague in 1912, but lapsed during the First World War. They were revived at conferences in Geneva in 1924 and 1925. It was at the 1925 conference that, even though cannabis was not on the agenda, the Egyptian delegate stated that hashish was at least as harmful as opium. He said it was: "…the principle cause of most of the cases of insanity occurring in Egypt," and should be included in the same narcotic category. Bizarrely, there were no objections, so controls were placed not only on the import and export of opium, but on cannabis.

The Demonising of cannabis

The Egyptian delegate's crusade was adopted by Harry J Anslinger who was appointed as the first Commissioner of the US Federal Bureau of Narcotics in 1930, a post he held for 32 years. Anslinger became fixated on cannabis and is credited as the man who single-handedly made marijuana illegal in the US, and by default, the rest of the world. This is not actually true as the drug was already subject to very strict controls thanks to the Geneva conference, but, Harry Anslinger, certainly played a significant role in demonising cannabis.

"Young people are slaves to this narcotic," he said in a radio address. "Their continuing addiction leads to mental deterioration, insanity and then they turn to violent crime and murder." Not only did Anslinger use the press but he also instigated anti-marijuana propaganda films including two, now infamous 1936 films. One is *Reefer Madness,* cautionary tales of high school students lured by pushers to try marijuana with dire and dreadful results, and *Marihuana,* with the tag line: 'Weird Orgies, Wild Parties and Unleashed Passions!'

Not only was violence inappropriately linked to marijuana but also to sexual promiscuity. By the end of 1936, the majority of US States had added marijuana to their most dangerous drugs list under the Uniform State Narcotic Acts, and the American public had the clear impression that marijuana was associated with crime, violence and wild sex. Given the increasing dominance of American culture, that view spread worldwide.

Some medics never gave up on it, like Pennsylvanian born psychiatrist Dr. Tod Hiro Mikuriya, (1839-1972) an outspoken advocate, and author of books like the *Marijuana Medical Papers;* information collected from the reference section at the National Library of Medicine in Maryland. Dr. Mikuriya prescribed medical cannabis to over 9,000 patients and founded The Society of Cannabis Clinicians, a non-profit and scientific society of qualified physicians and other professionals, dedicated to supporting medical cannabis use.

UN Single Convention on Narcotic Drugs 1961

Despite Dr. Mikuriya's best efforts, in the years after World War 2, cannabis was hardly used as a medicine. In the 1960s, it came to be thought of as a party drug rather than a therapy. As a recreational drug it induced either a calm, trance like state, or a euphoric, stimulated one. It also began to earn a reputation as an anti-establishment symbol associated with hippies and dropouts, so in 1961, was banned under the UN Single Convention on Narcotic Drugs.

This convention put cannabis in the most restrictive level of control and listed it in Schedules I and IV, alongside cocaine and opium. Cocaine and opium were viewed as being dangerous and easily abused and having extremely limited or no therapeutic value.

The countries that signed up to the United Nations' Convention principles had to go along with those restrictions and to the present day, many countries remain bound to the 1961 treaty.

While cannabis resin, extracts and tinctures, were all placed in restrictive categories, pure cannabidiol (CBD), was not Scheduled, meaning that with some country exceptions, CBD has remained a legal product and the industrial hemp industry continued to go about its business.

UK Misuse of Drugs Act 1971

All parties to the Single Convention were required to enact domestic legislation and enforce its requirements; this led to the 1971 Misuse of Drugs Act in the UK.

The Act provides a list of prohibited drugs, makes possession of these drugs unlawful and lays down further penalties not only for possession,

108

but for intent to supply. It creates three classes of controlled substances — A, B and C — and gives a range of penalties for illegal or unlicensed possession and supply within each class. Cannabis is still listed as a Class B drug under this Act, and the penalty in the UK for possession at Crown Court is up to five years with an unlimited fine. Possession with intent to supply in the Crown Court carries a prison sentence of up to 14 years with an unlimited fine, compared with up to 7 years for grievous bodily harm, or 2 years for causing death by dangerous driving.

In association with the Misuse of Drugs Act, came the Misuse of Drugs Regulations 2001, which placed controlled drugs in one of four Schedules. Until recently, cannabis was a Schedule 1 drug, along with coca leaf: the raw material for cocaine, raw opium and LSD, which means that it was deemed to have no medicinal value.

In July 2018, the UK government announced its intention to move: "...cannabis derived medicinal products..." into Schedule 2, which while still quite restrictive enables doctors to prescribe it in certain circumstances. This law change came into effect on 1 November 2018 and Cannabis now shares Schedule 2 with cocaine, diamorphine (a purified version of heroin used for pain), fentanyl (an opioid used for pain medication) and morphine (another opioid used to relieve pain). All of these drugs can kill; cannabis cannot.

In fact, almost 70 per cent of the peer reviewed studies done with medical cannabis between 1990 and 2014, came out in favour of cannabinoids as medicine, a signal to those able to change the law that it should be more readily available.

Regaining its place

Over the past 20 years, cannabis has slowly regained its status as an important medicine and therapy and is currently being used to treat conditions and illnesses where conventional medicine struggles.

CHAPTER 10

Cannabis: The Plant

Wild cannabis, sometimes known as feral cannabis or dickweed, grows over most of the world, generally in warm and humid climates. It is hardy and can be found high up in the Himalayas in Nepal, as well as in cooler and wetter regions like Canada and Northern Europe. It grows anywhere except for hot arid deserts, the Arctic and Antarctic. The main problem with wild cannabis is that it is less pure than the cultivated varieties grown in controlled conditions in greenhouses, or under cover.

Cannabis Varieties

Are there any major differences between cannabis sativa, indica and ruderalis? They look different. Sativa is tall, between 4 and 15 feet, with thin, long, pointy leaves, whereas indica is smaller, between 1 and 4 feet, with wider, shorter, more rounded leaves. Ruderalis is short, between 1 and 2 feet, and flowers automatically after about 3 to 4 weeks (auto-flowering), whereas the sativa and indica varieties need a change in sunlight hours to flower. Ruderalis is not often used in its pure form these days, probably because it has naturally low levels of THC.

Do the differences between the plants stop at their descriptions? In general, sativa strains produce a more stimulating, 'creative' and 'cerebral' effect, often followed by a desire to eat, known as the munchies by recreational users. Indica strains produce a more physical, relaxing or sedating effect, called couch lock by recreational users. Couch lock is when you're too relaxed to get off the sofa. A more important difference is the ratio of the two main compounds in cannabis. These are psychoactive tetrahydrocannabinol (THC) to non-psychoactive cannabidiol (CBD), as well as the proportions of the other minor cannabinoid compounds, terpenes (the aromatic oils that also have medical properties) and flavonoids (which give it its colour and have medical properties).

A quick guide to the cannabis plant

Cannabis plants can be male or female, or sometimes both (hermaphrodite). The female plants are used for medical cannabis and produce large flowers, rich in cannabinoids. The unfertilised female flower is called sinsemilla — from the Spanish 'without seeds.' To make sure most plants are female, growers clone the mother plant by taking a cutting and placing it in a growth medium. Once it has rooted, it can be grown into a mature plant genetically identical to the mother. Other parts of the plant do contain some cannabinoids, but in much smaller amounts. The leaves have concentrations of only 2 per cent to 3 per cent THC, while the unfertilised female flower has much higher concentrations, up to 16 per cent or so. The leaves — known as the trim — can be sold and used as a source of cannabinoids but have much lower monetary value. Other parts of the plant, such as the stem, the roots and the seeds contain very little cannabinoid.

Extraction

The first stage is drying and curing the flower, usually in an oven. This makes the extraction process easier, but the main reason is that the flower needs to go through a chemical process called decarboxylation. In their raw form, cannabinoids in the plant have an extra group of elements called a carboxyl ring. Cannabinoids that have not had that ring removed (by decarboxylation) do have some medicinal benefits but most benefit is found in the decarboxylated cannabinoids THC and CBD.

The non-decarboxylated cannabinoids are not intoxicating and it is for this reason that you can actually eat raw cannabis without any, or least not much, psychoactive effect. That carboxyl ring will disappear if the cannabis is 6 months old or older, or by heating it to about 120°C (250°F) for around 30 to 45 minutes. Then, the decarbed cannabinoids are ready to be extracted. There are many different ways of extracting the cannabinoids, terpenes and flavonoids.

Basically, the trichomes (hairs on the leaves) that contain most of the cannabinoids, need to be removed from the female flower. The resin covering the trichomes is sticky and is removed by rubbing your fingers over the bud. This is clearly not a satisfactory process for full-scale commercial production, so there are many different ways of extracting those medicinal cannabinoids and the other components of the plant.

At a non-industrial level, the dried bud can be sieved. The fine powder produced at the end of the sieving process is called 'Kief', which can be rolled and compressed into 'hash'. Another simple way of extracting the resin glands is by soaking the flower and leaf in iced water. The cold water breaks the glands away from the flower and leaf. The glands sink to the bottom of the container, because they are heavier than water, and the leaf and flower stay afloat and can be scooped away.

For industrial processes, the resin is usually removed by alcohol or butane or by "super-critical" carbon dioxide. The principle is simple, in that the resin dissolves into the oil or butane or CO_2 and, once separated, the oil or butane can be evaporated, leaving the cannabis oil behind.

The final cannabis oil is then usually, from a medicinal point of view, mixed with a carrier oil to be sold as the final product, either as capsule, an oil or as vaping fluid. Sometimes, it is important to know the carrier oil as some people can be allergic to it. The most usual carrier oil is palm kernel oil, or coconut oil, or another medium chain triglyceride (MCT), which is a partially man-made fat.

Cannabinoids are fat soluble, meaning they break down in fat and not in water and need a fatty oil to enable them to be carried into the body. The carrier oil also helps the bioavailability. Not all cannabis taken will be delivered to the circulation and the proportion absorbed is known as the bioavailability. Using MCT carrier oil will improve absorption and deliver more of the cannabinoids to your body's systems.

CHAPTER 11

Difference between hemp products and CBD products

Hemp

Many supplements you find in health food shops are labelled as hemp products rather than cannabis, but hemp is cannabis without the effects of THC.

Hemp, or industrial hemp as it's known in the trade, is the gentle cousin to cannabis; a variety of cannabis sativa that has very low, below 0.2 per cent, or even no THC, and relatively high CBD. It also contains very small amounts of other cannabinoids, as well as terpenes.

Hemp is legal in many countries because in most countries, THC must be below 0.2 per cent for the hemp product to be legal

China is emerging as a hemp 'superpower', holding over half the world's 600 product patents. Farmers in Europe — including the UK — and in parts of Asia and Canada, are allowed to grow it. Being a cannabis plant, it has often been lumped together with THC containing cannabis. In some countries, like most of the Middle East, growing hemp, even for industrial purposes is illegal.

It is an extremely versatile plant used in a huge variety of products like paper, shampoo, lotions, soap, biodiesel, plastics, paint, as well as to make clothes and rope. It can even be used to make a building material called hempcrete, and there's a bridge from sixth century Gaul made from it. It is also a very useful and nutritious food supplement, popular with vegetarians and vegans, and has received wide attention in the British media in recent months with *The Guardian* [lxxx] newspaper describing it as: "…a versatile raw material, that could once again become very lucrative." While the *Daily Mail* [lxxxi] described it as a "superfood." The *Mail* said: "The main health benefit of the hemp seed is that it is a complete protein and it has a rich source of omega 3. Omega 3, is widely known to reduce inflammation which often causes chronic illness."

The difference between hemp oil and CBD oil is that hemp oil is usually made by pressing the seeds of the plant, while CBD oil is mainly made from flowers and leaves. Hemp seeds contain very little, or even no cannabinoids, so pressing the them will not produce any THC or CBD.

As well as being high in omega 3, hemp oil also contains omega 6 polyunsaturated fats, and a useful range of minerals and vitamins; particularly vitamin E, vitamin B1, B2, potassium and magnesium. According to The Centre for Genetics, Nutrition and Health in Washington, US, hemp oil has a very well balanced 3:1 ratio of omega 6 to omega 3 essential fatty acids, which is described in nutrition literature as the optimal requirement for healthy human nutrition.

Excessive amounts of omega 6 polyunsaturated fatty acid are found in western diets. This is one of the underlying causes of many diseases, such as cardiovascular disease, cancer and inflammatory and autoimmune diseases. There is 15 to 16 times more omega 6 in western diets than there is omega 3, or a ratio of 15:1 to 16:1. This is one of the reasons westerners are vulnerable to heart disease, cancer, inflammatory and autoimmune diseases. If omega 6 can be reduced from 16 to 3, or 3:1, the reduction has a positive effect on a number of diseases, such as rheumatoid arthritis, asthma, and even some types of cancer. This makes hemp seed oil a useful nutritional supplement.

116

You can cook with its oil too, although usually not in high temperature cooking as it has quite a low smoking point, but it can be used the same way as olive oil, and in salad dressing, for example.

According to the American Academy of Dermatology, it is meant to be healthy for your skin and now many skin products, such as face creams, have hemp oil as the main ingredient. There are of course somewhat wilder claims of anti-aging benefits, but it does seem reasonable to suggest that hemp oil can benefit the skin, and at least help with skin disorders such as psoriasis, eczema, acne and dry skin. It has similar benefits for the hair and is now available in a number of hemp hair products, such as shampoos, oils and conditioners.

CBD Oils

CBD oil can be made from industrial hemp. In other chapters, we note the medical benefits of CBD, particularly its anti-anxiety effect, anti-epilepsy and painkilling properties.

Many manufacturers confuse the issue and market CBD oil as hemp oil, or even vice versa! There is nothing wrong with hemp oil, but it must be clearly labelled as different from its medicinal cousin, CBD oil, and from its other medicinal cousins, full extract cannabis oils which contain THC.

When buying CBD oil, note the ingredients listed on the packaging. Good products will be clearly labelled.

Good manufacturers are Endoca [lxxxii] and *Love CBD* [lxxxiii] in the UK and Europe, *Charlotte's Web* [lxxxiv] in the US and *Broken Coast* [lxxxv] in Canada. The United Patients Alliance, a British lobbying group, have a list of manufacturers they recommend [lxxxvi] and the US CBD Oil Review also makes many recommendations. [lxxxvii]

There are now attempts, in the UK, to regulate the market. As an example, the Cannabis Trades Association (CTA)[lxxxviii]. The CTA covers about 80 per cent of CBD producers selling products in the UK. They have tried to produce a standard of labelling. In the UK at least, it would be illegal to make medical claims for CBD so you will find CBD products that state: "This product is a food supplement and is not intended to diagnose, treat, cure or prevent any disease." We know CBD can treat some diseases but products in the UK and elsewhere cannot say so at the present time, as CBD has not been through the Medicines and Healthcare Products Regulatory (MHRA) safety check system. Manufacturers can only make medical claims if a product has been licensed by the MHRA.

There are other requirements for hemp products as the products are liable to the UK government's food labelling regulations. These are the name of the product; the 'best before' or 'use by date'; any necessary warnings; net quantity information; a list of ingredients if there is more than one; the name and address of the manufacturer, packer or seller; the country of origin if required; any special storage conditions and instructions for use. Packaging must also contain details of any allergens.

Sensible advice would be that if you want to use CBD for medicinal purposes you should only use a product that is clearly and understandably labelled.

Some CBD oil is marked as containing CBD and CBDA. This simply means that the product contains the acidic form of CBD — CBDAcid. This means that it is has not been fully decarboxylated and the original CBDA has not been converted fully to CBD. Some people prefer a mixture of CBD and CBDA rather than pure CBD. It is a matter of personal preference.

Most products, CBD oils or CBD/THC products available on the market, contain a whole range of other minor cannabinoids, albeit in very small doses. They also contain terpenes. These are called **full extract cannabis oils** and are different from pure CBD.

FURTHER READING

The Cannabis Grow Bible, The Definitive Guide to Growing Marijuana for Recreational and Medical Use by Greg Green Third Edition. Green Candy Press, San Francisco, 2017

The Cannabis Encyclopedia: The Definitive Guide to Cultivation and Consumption of Medical Marijuana by Jorge Cervantes. Van Patten Publishing, USA, 2015

The Endocannabinoid System: Genetics, Biochemistry, Brain Disorders and Therapy by Eric Murillo-Rodriguez. Elsevier London 2017

Handbook of Cannabis by Professor Roger G Pertwee. Oxford University Press, Oxford 2016

The Leafly Guide to Cannabis. A Handbook for the Modern Consumer by The Leafly Team. Twelve Hachette Book Group, New York, 2017. This is a user-friendly book, mainly designed for the recreational user is clearly written with helpful, practical tips.

Cannabis, motivation, and life satisfaction in an internet sample. *Substance Abuse Treatment and Prevention Policy,* 2006; **1**: 2 A paper by Barnwell SS, Earleywine M, Wilcox R. https://substanceabusepolicy.biomedcentral.com/articles/10.1186/1747-597X-1-2

If cannabis caused schizophrenia – how many cannabis users may need to be prevented in order to prevent one case of schizophrenia? England and Wales calculations. Addiction 2009; **104(11)**: 1856-61 A paper by Hickman M, Vickerman P, Macleod J, *et al.*

https://www.ncbi.nlm.nih.gov/pubmed/19832786

Cannabinoids for medical use: a systematic review and meta-analysis.
JAMA 2015; **313(24)**: 2456-73 A paper by Whiting PF, Wolff RF,
Deshpande S, *et al.*
https://www.ncbi.nlm.nih.gov/pubmed/26103030

*Australian Government Department of Health Therapeutic Goods
Administration, Medicinal Cannabis - Guidance Documents*, 2018.
Available from https://www.tga.gov.au/medicinal-cannabis-guidance-
documents.

*Health Products Regulatory Authority, Cannabis for Medical Use - A
Scientific Review*, 2017. Available at https://www.hpra.ie/docs/default-
source/publicationsforms/newsletters/cannabis-for-medical-use---a-
scientific-review.pdf?sfvrsn=7.

*National Academies of Sciences, Engineering and Medicine, The
Current State of Evidence and Recommendations for Research
Committee on the Health Effects of Marijuana: An Evidence Review and
Research Agenda*, 2017. A report from the National Academies of
Sciences, Engineering, Medicine. Available at
https://www.nap.edu/read/24625/chapter/1#xii.

*Systematic Review: efficacy and safety of medical marijuana in selected
neurologic disorders: report of the Guideline Development
Subcommittee of the American Academy of Neurology. Neurology*
2014; 82: 1556-1563. A paper by Koppel BS, Brust JCM, Fife T et al.
https://www.ncbi.nlm.nih.gov/pubmed/24778283

Report of Dame Sally Davies, Chief Medical Officer, contains a number of broad generic academic references which may be useful https://www.gov.uk/government/publications/cannabis-scheduling-review-part-1

Report to the All Party Parliament Group on Drug Policy Reform by myself and my daughter, Dr. Jennifer Barnes, a clinical psychologist – freely available on line at https://www.drugpolicyreform.net/ or through the End Our Pain website (https://endourpain.org/). Contains over 200 references to the literature on all subjects.

UK Home Office website contains a number of recent publications on cannabis including the current guidance https://www.gov.uk/government/collections/medicinal-cannabis-information-and-resources

Cannabinoids for medical use: a systematic review and meta-analysis. *JAMA* **2015**; 313: 2456-2473. A paper by Whiting PF, Wolff RF, Deshpande S et al. https://www.ncbi.nlm.nih.gov/pubmed/26103030

World Health Organization Expert Committee on Drug Dependence, Cannabidiol (CBD) Critical Review Report, 2018. Available at https://www.who.int/medicines/access/controlled-substances/CannabidiolCriticalReview.pdf.

And further cannabis review at: https://www.who.int/medicines/access/controlled-substances/Cannabis_Review_QA_26July2018.pdf?ua=1

UK Advocate / Lobbying Groups
CLEAR — https://www.clear-uk.org

End Our Pain — https://endourpain.org

Families4access — www.families4access.com

United Patients Alliance — https://www.upalliance.org

Medical Cannabis Clinicians Society -- https://www.ukmccs.org

US and Canada Recommended Manufacturers

CBD Oil Review — https://cbdoilreview.org/cbd-companies

Many other groups from different countries are available online. As usual with the internet, be selective about what you find online.

REFERENCES AND LINKS

NOTE: This is a small selection of the papers available on the free website PubMed

CHAPTER 1

[i] 25 per cent stop taking opioids:
https://www.statnews.com/2018/04/02/marijuana-legal-opioid-prescriptions/
[ii] Centers for Disease Control: https://www.theguardian.com/us-news/2018/aug/16/us-drug-overdose-deaths-opioids-fentanyl-cdc
[iii] Office for National Statistics prescription drug deaths:
https://www.ons.gov.uk/peoplepopulationandcommunity/birthsdeathsandmarriages/deaths/bulletins/deathsrelatedtodrugpoisoninginenglandandwales/2017registrations
[iv] Brazillian Researchers 2011:
https://www.nature.com/articles/npp20116
[v] University of Milan, Italy 2012:
https://www.ncbi.nlm.nih.gov/pmc/articles/PMC3579246/
[vi] Molecular Therapeutics Journal, 2011:
http://mct.aacrjournals.org/content/early/2011/05/10/1535-7163.MCT-10-1100.short
[vii] National Institute of Mental Health, 2000:
https://www.royalqueenseeds.com/blog-the-antioxidant-properties-of-cbd-n1061
[viii] Journal of Experimental Medicine, 2012:
http://jem.rupress.org/content/209/6/1121
[ix] University of South Carolina 2009:
https://www.ncbi.nlm.nih.gov/pmc/articles/PMC2828614/

[x] National Institutes of Mental Health, Bethesda, Maryland 1998: https://www.ncbi.nlm.nih.gov/pmc/articles/PMC20965/

[xi] University of Naples 2013: https://www.ncbi.nlm.nih.gov/pubmed/23415610

[xii] University of Eastern Piedmont, 28100 Novara, Italy 2008: https://www.ncbi.nlm.nih.gov/pubmed/18681481

[xiii] Complutense University, Madrid, 28040, Spain 2015: https://www.ncbi.nlm.nih.gov/pubmed/25252936

[xiv] University of Naples 2015: https://www.ncbi.nlm.nih.gov/pubmed/26197538

[xv] 2014: https://www.ncbi.nlm.nih.gov/pubmed/25269802

[xvi] University of Lodz, Poland 2008: https://www.ncbi.nlm.nih.gov/pubmed/19112869

[xvii] Hokuriku University, Kanazawa, Japan 1995: https://www.ncbi.nlm.nih.gov/pubmed/7728937

[xviii] Journal of Neuroscience 2002: http://www.jneurosci.org/content/22/11/4720.full

[xix] Journal of Immunology 2005: https://www.jni-journal.com/article/S0165-5728(05)00160-8/abstract

[xx] University of Eastern Piedmont, Novara, Italy 2008: https://pubs.acs.org/doi/full/10.1021/np8002673

[xxi] Endocannabinoid Research Group, Institute of Biomolecular Chemistry - Pozzuoli, Napoli, Italy 2013: https://www.ncbi.nlm.nih.gov/pubmed/23941747

[xxii] G W Pharmaceuticals: https://www.gwpharm.com/

CHAPTER 3

[xxiii] Drug Policy Reform 2011: https://www.drugpolicyreform.net/

[xxiv] Universities of São Paulo, South and Santa Catarina and other Brazilian institutions 2011: https://www.ncbi.nlm.nih.gov/pmc/articles/PMC3079847/

[xxv] Dame Sally Davies review 2018, https://www.gov.uk/government/publications/cannabis-scheduling-review-part-1

[xxvi] National Academies of Sciences, Engineering and Medicine in the US 2017: http://www.nationalacademies.org/hmd/Reports/2017/health-effects-of-cannabis-and-cannabinoids.aspx

[xxvii] McGill University, Montreal, Canada, 2018: https://www.mcgill.ca/maxbellschool/channels/news/safe-cannabis-pain-relief-without-high-291089

[xxviii] Nature Neuroscience, appetite 2014: https://www.nature.com/articles/nn.3647

[xxix] Wright State University School of Medicine, Portland, Ohio, US 2014 https://www.ncbi.nlm.nih.gov/pubmed/25337447

[xxx] Universities of South Santa Catarina and Santa Catarina in Brazil 2018: https://www.ncbi.nlm.nih.gov/pubmed/30087591

[xxxi] Oregon Health and Science University, and the Veterans Affairs Health Care System in Portland, Oregan, US 2017 https://www.ncbi.nlm.nih.gov/pubmed/28806794

[xxxii] Palo Alto University 2017: https://www.ncbi.nlm.nih.gov/pubmed/28349316 https://www.cannabisclinics.ca/doctors-in-canada/

[xxxiii] Neuroscience Research Australia 2017: https://www.ncbi.nlm.nih.gov/pmc/articles/PMC5289988/

[xxxiv] Skaggs Institute for Chemical Biology, California, US 2006: https://www.ncbi.nlm.nih.gov/pubmed/17140265

[xxxv] Sunnybrook Health Sciences Centre, University of Toronto, Canada 2018: https://www.nbcnews.com/health/health-news/cannabis-drug-eases-agitation-alzheimer-s-patients-n894111

xxxvi Journal of General Practice 2017:

https://www.omicsonline.org/open-access/comedication-with-cannabidiol-may-slow-down-the-progression-of-motorneuron-disease-a-case-report-2329-9126-1000316.php?aid=91246&view=mobile

xxxvii Harbor-UCLA Medical Centre, Torrance, US 2014:

https://www.ncbi.nlm.nih.gov/pubmed/25264643

xxxviii The University of Miami Miller School of Medicine, The Miami Project to Cure Paralysis, Miami, US, Scythian Biosciences, Toronto Canada, 2018: https://physician-news.umiamihealth.org/concussion-pill-shows-promise-in-pre-clinical-pilot-study/

xxxix American Cancer Society: https://www.cancer.org/cancer/cancer-basics/lifetime-probability-of-developing-or-dying-from-cancer.html

xl Cancer UK, survival rates: https://www.cancerresearchuk.org/health-professional/cancer-statistics/survival/common-cancers-compared

xli Cancer UK Survival rates: https://www.cancerresearchuk.org/health-professional/cancer-statistics/survival/common-cancers-compared

xlii Journal of National Cancer Institute, 1975:

https://www.ncbi.nlm.nih.gov/pubmed/1159836

xliii University of Wisconsin, Wisconsin, UK 2005:

https://www.ncbi.nlm.nih.gov/pubmed/15753356

xliv University of Otago, Dunedin, New Zealand 2009:

https://www.ncbi.nlm.nih.gov/pubmed/19442435

xlv Central Drug Research Institute, Lucknow, India and Department of Pathology at Ohio State University, Columbus, Ohio, US, 2014:

https://www.ncbi.nlm.nih.gov/pubmed/25115386

xlvi G W Pharmaceuticals 2017:

https://www.gwpharm.com/about/news/gw-pharmaceuticals-achieves-positive-results-phase-2-proof-concept-study-glioma

xlvii St George's brain cancer 2104:

https://www.ncbi.nlm.nih.gov/pubmed/25398831

xlviii Complutense University brain cancer 2011:

https://www.nature.com/articles/6603236

xlix St George's Hospital, London, UK:

https://www.sgul.ac.uk/research/research-news/cannabis-extract-can-have-dramatic-effect-on-brain-cancer-says-new-research

l World Health Organisation depression:

https://www.who.int/mental_health/management/depression/wfmh_paper_depression_wmhd_2012.pdf

li United Patients' Alliance: https://www.upalliance.org/medical-information/medical-evidence

lii Dalhousie University, Halifax 2016:

https://www.ncbi.nlm.nih.gov/pmc/articles/PMC4737462/

liii Ethan Russo, Neuroendocrinology Letters, endocannabinoid deficiency syndrome 2004:

https://www.researchgate.net/profile/Ethan_Russo/publication/2750323 77_Russo_Clinical_Endocannabinoid_Deficiency_NEL_2004/links/552f d5af0cf27acb0de7c158/Russo-Clinical-Endocannabinoid-Deficiency-NEL-2004.pdf?origin=publication_list

liv University of São Paulo, Brazil 2014:

https://www.ncbi.nlm.nih.gov/pubmed/25237116

lv University of São Paulo, Brazil 2018:

https://www.ncbi.nlm.nih.gov/pmc/articles/PMC5958190/

lvi University of Milan, Italy 2018:

https://www.ncbi.nlm.nih.gov/pubmed/29789034

https://www.marijuanadoctors.com/

lvii Hannover Medical School, Hannover, Germany 2017:

https://www.ncbi.nlm.nih.gov/pmc/articles/PMC5447929/

https://www.ncbi.nlm.nih.gov/pmc/articles/PMC5578129/

CHAPTER 4

[lviii] United Patients Alliance (UPA) recommended manufacturers: https://www.upalliance.org/newsmediainternal/2017/5/3/cbd-rich-hemp-products

[lix] CBD Oil Review: https://cbdoilreview.org/cbd-companies/

[lx] Just CBD Store: https://www.justcbdstore.com/product/signature-cbd-cartridges-northern-lights/

[lxi] Koi CBD: https://koicbd.com/shop/cbd-vape-devices/

[lxii] Dank Vapes: https://www.dankvapes.co.uk/collections/vaporizers

[lxiii] SpeedWeed: https://www.speedweed.com/?v=79cba1185463

[lxiv] Hemp Elf: https://hempelf.com/collections/edibles

[lxv] Psychology Today 2011: https://www.psychologytoday.com/us/blog/all-about-sex/201105/marijuana-and-sex-surprising-results-blogger-s-informal-survey

CHAPTER 5

[lxvi] University of Colorado, Colorado, US 2018: https://www.denverhealth.org/-/media/denver-health-marijuana--pregnancy-study.pdf?la=en&hash=7CF1182B6937B9E4267378A1E5F04D8ED221DC6C

[lxvii] European and American scientists 2015: https://www.ncbi.nlm.nih.gov/pubmed/26103030

[lxviii] Journal Anesthesiology, 2018: http://anesthesiology.pubs.asahq.org/article.aspx?articleid=2674297

[lxix] National Health Service (NHS) cannabis 2018: https://www.nhs.uk/conditions/medical-cannabis/

lxx Journal, Human Molecular Genetics, 2017:

https://academic.oup.com/hmg/article/26/13/2462/3574683

lxxi University of Bristol, Bristol, UK 2009:

https://www.ncbi.nlm.nih.gov/pubmed/19832786

lxxii The Lancet, 2007:

https://www.thelancet.com/journals/lancet/article/PIIS0140-
6736(07)60464-4/fulltext?refuid=S0006-3223%2812%2900685-
3&refissn=0006-3223

lxxiii American Psychiatric Association (APA):

https://www.psychiatry.org/psychiatrists/practice/dsm

lxxiv The Scripps Institute, La Jolla, California, US 2011:

https://www.ncbi.nlm.nih.gov/pubmed/21321675

lxxv University of Pennsylvania, Philadelphia, US 2018:

https://jamanetwork.com/journals/jamapsychiatry/article-
abstract/2678214

https://actionnetwork.org/user_files/user_files/000/022/633/original/2018
_JAMA_cognition_review.pdf?link_id=1&can_id=4dd1926dc59aae056e
a65db4ca82244e&source=email-jama-meta-analysis-cannabis-
exposure-not-associated-with-residual-adverse-impact-on-cognitive-
performance&email_referrer=email_338205&email_subject=jama-meta-
analysis-cannabis-exposure-not-associated-with-residual-adverse-
impact-on-cognitive-performance

lxxvi Sativex study 2012: https://www.mstrust.org.uk/research/research-
updates/update120815-longer-term-use-sativex-risks-and-benefits

CHAPTER 7

lxxvii Dame Sally Davies review of cannabis 2018:

https://www.gov.uk/government/publications/cannabis-scheduling-
review-part-1

lxxviii Wikipedia legality of cannabis:

https://en.wikipedia.org/wiki/Legality_of_cannabis

lxxix Supplements in review: https://supplementsinreview.com/blog/is-cbd-legal-in-my-country-global-guide-to-cbd-legality/

PART 2

CHAPTER 11

lxxx The Guardian: https://www.theguardian.com/society/2018/jun/11/the-hemp-revival-why-marijuanas-cousin-could-soon-be-big-business
lxxxi Daily Mail: https://www.dailymail.co.uk/femail/article-4787782/Is-hemp-going-new-super-food.html
lxxxii Endoca: https://www.endoca.com/en-gb
lxxxiii Love CBD: https://www.lovecbd.org/
lxxxiv Charlotte's Web: https://www.cwhemp.com/
lxxxv Broken Coast: https://www.brokencoastrx.com/
lxxxvi UPI: https://www.upalliance.org/newsmediainternal/2017/5/3/cbd-rich-hemp-products
lxxxvii CBD Oil Review: https://cbdoilreview.org/cbd-companies/
lxxxviii Cannabis Trades Association: https://cannabistrades.uk/

OTHER REFERENCES
THC

McGill University: https://www.mcgill.ca/newsroom/channels/news/safe-cannabis-pain-relief-without-high-291089
anti-inflammatory, immune suppression:
https://www.ncbi.nlm.nih.gov/pmc/articles/PMC4885748/
pain relief: https://www.nhs.uk/news/neurology/cannabis-for-nerve-pain-studied/
antioxidant: https://www.ncbi.nlm.nih.gov/pubmed/10863546

CBD

Anti-anxiety: https://www.ncbi.nlm.nih.gov/pubmed/20829306

anti-cancer: https://www.ncbi.nlm.nih.gov/pubmed/22506672

breast cancer: http://mct.aacrjournals.org/content/10/7/1161.long

antioxidant and neuroprotective: https://echoconnection.org/cbd-has-antioxidant-and-neuroprotective-properties-what-does-that-mean/

pain: https://www.ncbi.nlm.nih.gov/pmc/articles/PMC5569620/

Myrcene

Anti-cancer: https://thetruthaboutcancer.com/phytochemicals-tree-essential-oils/

Limonene

Anti-stress and anxiety:

https://www.ncbi.nlm.nih.gov/pubmed/12499653

Japanese psychiatrists: https://www.karger.com/Article/Abstract/96889

anti-cancer: https://www.ncbi.nlm.nih.gov/pmc/articles/PMC5894671/

anti-inflammatory: https://www.ncbi.nlm.nih.gov/pubmed/28260017

Caryophyllene

pain: https://www.ncbi.nlm.nih.gov/pubmed/24210682

anticancer: https://www.ncbi.nlm.nih.gov/pubmed/18053325

mood enhancer: https://www.ncbi.nlm.nih.gov/pubmed/24930711

anti-inflammatory: http://bone.imedpub.com/antiarthritic-and-anti-inflammatory-activity-of-beta-caryophyllene-against-freunds-complete-adjuvant-induced-arthritis-in-wistar-rats.php?aid=7220

anti-arthritis: http://bone.imedpub.com/antiarthritic-and-anti-inflammatory-activity-of-beta-caryophyllene-against-freunds-complete-adjuvant-induced-arthritis-in-wistar-rats.php?aid=7220

Linalool

anti-anxiety: https://www.ncbi.nlm.nih.gov/pubmed/19962290

anti-convulsant: https://www.ncbi.nlm.nih.gov/pubmed/10374249

anti-acne: https://www.goodguide.com/ingredients/512321-linalool-ingredient-information-reviews#/

Flavonoids

Quecertin: https://europepmc.org/abstract/med/10869101

Beta-sitosterol: anti-inflammatory:

https://www.ncbi.nlm.nih.gov/pmc/articles/PMC5411862/

Cannflavin: anti-inflammatory:

https://www.ncbi.nlm.nih.gov/pmc/articles/PMC4885748/

Printed in Great Britain
by Amazon